Personal Care Handbook

Survival Beyond The Caregiver

GLORIA LOPEZ

Order this book online at www.trafford.com
or email orders@trafford.com

Most Trafford titles are also available at major online book retailers.

Print information available on the last page.

ISBN: 978-1-4907-7284-4 (sc)
ISBN: 978-1-4907-7285-1 (e)

Library of Congress Control Number: 2016906646

Trafford rev. 09/12/2017

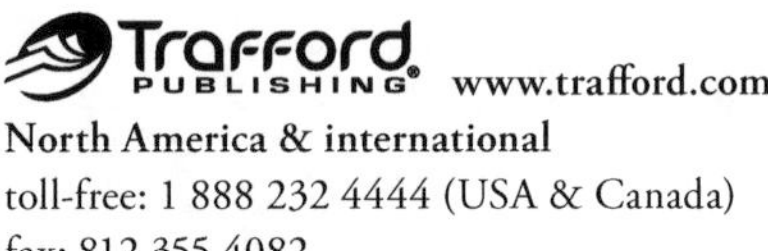

www.trafford.com

North America & international
toll-free: 1 888 232 4444 (USA & Canada)
fax: 812 355 4082

Contents

Special Thanks

My son Michael, without whom I would have had the experiences that led to my understanding of the importance of documenting daily information, and

Debra Butler for her continued assistance and recommendation through her personal experiences of the importance of documentation.

ଓଃ ଓଃ ଓଃ ଓଃ

About the Author

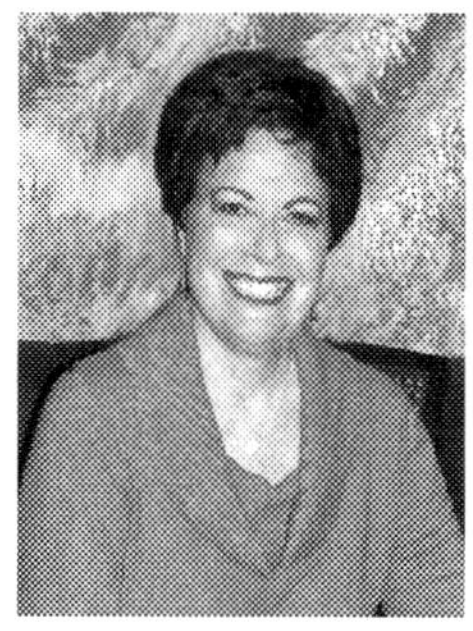

For over forty-one years, Gloria A. Lopez has worked with children with disabilities and their families and with adults who were diagnosed with medical conditions later in life.

A mother of three children, her son was born with a disability—Spina Bifida. Her experiences led her to design books that offer an individual self-empowerment by taking a more active role in their medical care through documentation.

As a parent of a young adult with multiple anomalies since birth, the challenges presented by the professionals involved and the many changes in the health condition as well as the transitional evolution to an adult provided the purpose for the development of this book and the hope that if a transfer of care was necessary, there would be a minimal break in the daily care with the medical information provided. It has ensured the continuity of the health of her son. The record keeping from a caregiver has provided invaluable information when a medical situation arose, being available to share the information with the medical team assisting with the diagnosis.

Ms. Lopez believes that documenting your medical history and daily care will help prevent and minimize medical errors and assist the medical team. She is a speaker and an advocate on the purpose of documentation and has authored *Personal Medical Journal*, *My Personal Medical Journal*, *Personal Medical Pocket Journal*, *Personal Caregivers Handbook*, and the *Personal Care Handbook.*

Personal Care Handbook

by

Gloria A. Lopez

The *Personal Care Handbook* is designed to provide an overview of an individual's medical history by having complete information, documented diagnosis history, mobility issues or disability, explaining the purpose of their medical needs in the event there is a change of the primary caregiver, hence "survival beyond the caregiver."

It can give the individual with special needs the empowerment of independence. Should the primary caregiver change, there would be a continuity of care because the medical needs are documented. It also provides the individual, parent, spouse, caregiver, and professional the opportunity to have the most pertinent personal information to best care for the individual throughout their lifetime.

Having the need for someone to assist with daily care or to ensure the continuity of health is difficult. There are many ways a person can ensure such continuity, and one is having all the documented medical information in an easily accessible location.

Ms. Lopez started this book when she realized that her son, born with a disability and requiring the assistance of others to ensure his continuity of health, needed to organize his medical information and daily care into an easy-to-use system. Since she had the majority of the information in her head or on papers in different locations, she decided it was best to organize the information into a central format explaining to him their purpose so he will know; if it was necessary one day, he could survive should something happen to her. She also found out that the information made it easier when she used various service agencies, Medicaid/Medi-Cal or state program, insurance, legal, and many other service providers, especially if some type of funding program was available. The information made it easy not only to recall data but also to produce copies of reports that have occurred over his lifetime.

By producing the data requested, it provided the review committee to accept many times the application as an example within four (4) days instead of the normal two to four months. Over the years, much of the information had been discarded by the professional, hospital, school, and service agency used. Therefore, it was important to have the data available not only to best assist with the application but also to expedite the outcome.

The records that begin at the onset of the diagnosis are papers, reports, X-rays, and tests that needed to be recorded and copied for future use; and you may want to have different applications depending on the data—a binder or file with all the surgical or medical reports, another for any legal or social service documentation, etc.

There are sectioned categories depending on the various needs required. This is YOUR *Personal Care Handbook*, and the format presented is to assist you. The important thing to remember is that this handbook is to be tailored to the individual's needs. There are no two individuals alike; therefore, complete the forms and tailor the data by editing and adding information.

Please remember:

- Keep all data and information in lay terms, not in professional terminology that will make it difficult to read and follow, so anyone can understand.
- The information supplied should be kept in strict confidence for the individual and whoever they want to read the handbook.
- It will be important to be honest and provide essential information so the caregiver will be able to care for the individual.
- There will be information within this book that you may not need, and that will be to your discretion.
- Feel free to add data to best assist you.

To aid further with health management, ask the physician, dentist, and any medical professional for a copy of their report for your files. This can include the following: copies of any X-rays, laboratory studies, special procedures, surgical, and special testing reports. Add any information that you feel is pertinent or will be helpful to another physician, therapist, or a service provider. You can place this information in a separate binder.

Purchase dividers and a three-ring binder from the local supermarket, office supply store, or pharmacy to create the personal health care binder. It will make it easier for you to locate information by using dividers sectioned into the different disciplines or fields of service from which you are working (i.e., neurosurgery, surgical, X-ray, psychological, physician summaries, laboratory results, and school reports such as the Individualized Educational Program (IEP), etc.

It is suggested that you request copies of X-ray films (i.e., an actual film copy) and their reports for the permanent health records. They will be useful as a comparison and provide the necessary information needed for treatment. It can prove to be invaluable. To store these copies, you will find that they fit perfectly into an art portfolio that is available at your local art supply store.

You may also want a copy of all X-rays in a different format. Ask the medical facility for the formats they have available (i.e., photo printout, a soft copy such as a USB flash drive, DVD, etc.) to make it easy for you to carry and store. Find out what is compatible with your computer and the computer at the medical facility requesting a copy. It is beneficial that you have the pertinent information with you when visiting various doctors and when traveling. Remember, a USB flash drive or DVD may not always be accessible by another medical facility so take your binders and printed information for backup.

If you or the individual you care for has special needs and require caregivers, produce a video showing the required assistance. Be sure to include feeding, bathing, cooking, transfer techniques, and personal care. This gives security to you and the caregiver knowing how best to provide the needed care.

Explain in the video:

- The medical condition, by showing literature, illustrations, or the X-ray films. (If they are available, you can tape them to a window that allows light to filter through and explain the medical situation.)
- Always maintain the dignity of the individual to be cared for, therefore always clothed when shown in various techniques and processes needed.
- Daily care, showing where items need to be located in the kitchen, bathroom, and the rest of the house. If the individual has a mobility disability, show how and where to place items within their reach, such as dishes, glasses, cooking items, daily care, towels, etc.
  - ✓ Remember, a person with a visual disability works on memorization; therefore, it is important to keep household items, clothing, furniture, etc., as originally placed.
  - ✓ A person in a wheelchair needs items lowered to be able to reach independently in their home.
- All supplies, medical and any special items, should be shown to them and discussed on what they are, how to use them, and care for their cleaning. Express any areas of concern that require specific attention (i.e., ostomy care, lymphedema wraps, CPAP type machine, respirator, etc.).
- Instructions that are crucial to the situation, which may include incontinence and wound care or specific attention with frequency as needed.
- How to use any equipment and the maintenance required. Describe in detail how to do transfers from one piece of equipment to another, into or out of other furnishings such as wheelchairs, walkers, etc., while sitting, lying down, when at home or when out in the community, including when traveling.

- Mobility and transportation—how to transport, what are the local services available, how to be secured while being transported and the equipment used (i.e., wheelchairs, walkers, etc.), circumstances for special consideration, equipment for daily and long-distance trips, and air travel (i.e., breakdown and securing equipment and how to use lifts and ramps, etc.).
- In traveling, show what supplies to use, the necessary equipment, and the care required while away from home.

This video recording will help to provide continuity of care to enhance the quality of life, furthering the feeling of security that the individual will be taken care of if the main caregiver is no longer available.

Your handbook should have dividers to contain information regarding the following:

a. Educational material that helps explain the disability and how it affects the end user.
b. Pictures that help explain the disability or a particular situation. These can be available online or through an organization that specializes in a specific area.
c. Information if cognitive areas are involved and how a person can learn.
d. List of support groups, educational programs, or conferences that can be available through a specific organization.
e. As much resourceful information you have or where it can be obtained, online, the library, through a local, state, or national organization. There may be several different groups that can give needed assistance especially to a person who is taking over the care of an individual with special needs.
f. A contact list of services, phone numbers, contact information if available, Web address, and the type of services offered or that you are using.
g. Educational school programs, medical programs and services, anything that will benefit you and the individual with special needs in order to maintain a continuity of services and health.

Check with your specific insurance program if the hospital facility has a genetics department that offers support, and follow up on your specific diagnosis, such as a Spina Bifida Clinic or Cerebral Palsy Clinic, etc. Many of these clinics work with children, but some of them will include adults. They offer a wealth of services and can be extremely helpful. They may also work with your primary physicians therefore giving you an additional medical support team available.

The difficulty can be when an individual becomes eighteen years of age and many of the support programs once offered are no longer available and you may feel like you have been dropped off the center of the earth. It takes some research to locate a physician team and the necessary support needed to maintain a continuity of health. Check with your local university or medical teaching centers to see if they can offer the medical support you may need. As well, you will need to see what funding programs can be helpful in providing assistance.

Some of the support and funding programs require information even as far back as infancy for acceptance into their program when working as an adult at <u>any age</u>. Ms. Lopez has been witness to a situation where a family member with medical issues that require daily monitoring and assistance is in his late sixties and has been under the care of his mother for his entire life. The mother is getting on with age, and the siblings are trying to get program funding and services to help their brother. Because he was not in the various programs available in his earlier years, they must supply information back to his childhood, which has been very difficult to locate. This caused problems in being accepted into various programs, as well as to understand all that is needed to care for their brother. If there had been a file or some type of information in the family files, it would have been easier, especially in a time they are also dealing with the issues of the parent.

You may want to check with a legal advisor to discuss which legal documents to consider for your loved one. Inquire how to protect their assets, that include the advantages and the disadvantages. Understand their importance, why they are needed, the procedures required, the financial costs, and any other questions or concerns so you can be informed of the options available. The following are some documents to consider:

1. Emancipated Child vs. Unemancipated Child. A child can be discharged or remain dependent regarding the care from their parent. Discuss how this affects the individual when they are over the age of eighteen (18) years, and the various funding and service programs available.
2. Special Needs Trust. An irrevocable trust in which the disabled beneficiary's assets are protected to remain eligible to the various funding and services available.
3. Conservatorship. A guardian or a protector is appointed to manage the financial and/or daily life of another due to a physical or mental limitation or old age. If you have a Special Needs Trust discuss the appropriate conservatorship to consider one or both of the following:
    a. If only for medical. Generally, if you manage the Special Needs Trust this may be all you will need, but discuss this with your legal advisor.
    b. If a financial is needed. Be sure to discuss the meaning and the procedure when needing to obtain funds.
4. Advanced Health Directive. A document that makes provisions for health care decisions in the event the person becomes incompetent to make such a decision.

5. Power of Attorney. Written authorization to represent or act on another's behalf to make decisions if the signer is unable to make such decisions.
6. Any other legal venue in your state or country to consider in order to protect your loved one.

This is especially important if your loved one is over the age of eighteen (18) years. It allows anyone to share or discuss information with you from one or more of the following services: a healthcare service provider, the medical team, during a doctor visit, while in the hospital, or with various social service agencies.

It is important to contact your current program providers of any changes especially should there be a change in the primary caregiver or a move to a new location outside the area you are receiving services. Be sure to ask what is the procedure, and the appropriate paperwork or documents required to insure there is a continuum of service. This will assist to make an easier transition, and, especially helpful for the new person who is handling all the paperwork.

Therefore it is important to keep all of your files in a location that is easy to access for anyone who may need to take over the responsibility of caring for your loved one or yourself.

There are several sections to this handbook. I have provided you with forms to use as guidelines. You can customize them to your needs with the digital copy that is available online at www.LCPBooks.com or by contacting our office at info@lcpbooks.com.

Ms. Lopez has published the *Personal Caregiver Handbook* that has forms customized for the individual with special needs who requires the assistance of a caregiver. This not only helps give guidance and instructions for what is needed in the daily care, but it also provides the primary caregiver and the individual who requires the assistance the assurance that everything has been done daily. Also, should a medical situation occur, it will allow the caregiver to document what happened should medical assistance be needed. More information on how to obtain this handbook and other publications is available on the back of this handbook.

Consider this *Personal Care Handbook* as a tool to assist you. There will no longer be a need to memorize every detail regarding the medical history, helping to eliminate the redundancy of information. The health care professional would be pleased to know that you have your information organized. This will help contribute to optimum care.

Remember, *Personal Care Handbook* preprinted forms have a copyright, and unauthorized distribution is illegal.

Congratulations! You now have the comfort of accuracy and assistance with the daily personal care and monitoring needed.

Enjoy the peace of mind!

✧ ✧ ✧

The Primary Caregiver

The love of caring for an individual is supreme and spiritual in nature. It brings light, balance, love, friendship, and a continuity of health. It is relentless, yet the feeling of knowing you are helping an individual live a life filled with the abundance intended is gratifying. For the slightest smile and the lightest touch can bring warmth to the simplest of tasks, a gift offered to another individual.

Today, knowing that even though one person may know how to care properly for another person, you can provide information so another person can be entrusted to handle the care needed in the event a change of a caregiver is necessary. The importance is directed to the individual who requires assistance who will know that they can be cared for appropriately without a major break in their care.

A caregiver is the peace offered an individual who requires some special assistance. It offers the peace of not being alone and helps to eliminate the fears of living daily trying to get through the simplest of tasks. However, it is not easy for either the caregiver or the recipient for both need to find the balance in the care and needs to be met with respect and honor to each other. Having a system to follow makes it easier in many ways but does not account for the total picture that includes the personalities involved, gentleness, and the patience required with each other.

By designing the *Personal Care Handbook*, or, as I also call it, "Survival Beyond the Caregiver," hope is given that if it was necessary to transfer care to another individual, at least the health history information would not be lost and they would not have to start over. It offers a peace of mind. It will take some time to gather the information, but in small amounts of time, it can be gathered to help you and the next person to care for your loved one.

Forms List

The supplied forms within each area give you example guidelines. It will be important for you to customize each area to ensure that all needs are met by adding pertinent information as this is the individual's personalized handbook.

You can also request a disc or a USB copy of the forms in order to assist you in tailoring them to meet your needs or go online to www.LCPBooks.com and download a copy for a minimal fee.

The caregiver needs to understand the importance of all the forms being completed daily.

1. **Alerts and Concerns Log**
    a. It is important to list any medical, physical, or emotional areas of concern that requires attention.
    b. Keep updated as situations arise.

2. **Allergy List**
    a. This is important to keep up to date and include all allergies, such as foods, medication, herbal supplements, environmental, etc.

3. **Caregiver**
    This area is meant to assist the individual who will require a caregiver to assist with daily home care and the primary caregiver who is seeking assistance and who provides information on how to hire a caregiver, an interview sheet, and instructions once you have hired a caregiver or service.
    a. Caregiver Agreement
    b. Caregiver Daily Checklist
    c. Caregiver Employment Application
    d. Caregiver Guidelines
    e. Caregiver Hire Guidelines
    f. Caregiver Interview Checklist
    g. Caregiver Interview Evaluation
    h. Caregiver Interview Guidelines
    i. Caregiver Interview Questionnaire
    j. Caregiver Job Description

4. **Chart Notes**
    a. Use this form to leave a note regarding an occurrence, medical concern, or as a daily update.
    b. This will alert any other caregiver on a situation that has occurred or requires monitoring.

5. **Community Transportation**
    a. Guidelines to assist with mobility instructions for any form of community transportation: bus, train, muni, rapid transit system, etc.
    b. Feel free to customize it to meet your needs.

6. **Emergency Contact Information**
    a. The individual or the primary caregiver needs to complete this information.
    b. Make a copy and post it on a cabinet or refrigerator for easy access.

7. **Equipment Maintenance**
    a. Sample form showing how to use, care for, and precautions for any equipment that is utilized.
    b. Separate fill-in section of this form for you to customize to meet your needs.
    c. Be sure to add all equipment and the specific needs for its care.

8. **Home Care Facilities and Independent Living**
    a. Budget and Independent Living Needs
    b. Home Care Questionnaire
    c. Independent Living Property Search

9. **Medical Concerns Checklist**
    a. When an illness or medical condition occurs, this section describes how the caregiver can best assist the individual. It is also helpful for the medical team when an emergency arises.
    b. It will be important that all information is thoroughly documented and kept up to date.
    c. Separate fill-in section of this form for you to customize to meet your needs.

10. **Medical Occurrence Log**
    a. This form is used when a medical condition occurs to keep everyone abreast of a situation.

b. To prevent future confusion, use one form per type of medical situation. This will maintain an independent frequency log of reoccurring events, such as urinary tract infections (UTIs), seizures, falls, etc.
c. Keep additional copies available in the back of the binder.

11. Medication Daily Schedule/Medication Chart Schedule

a. This is VERY IMPORTANT to keep up to date especially when medication needs to be distributed by the caregiver.
b. Keep a copy with the medication bottles.

12. Personal Bag Organization

a. Quick reference for any items needed when leaving the home.

13. Personal Medical Summary

Summarize all past and current health information.

a. If you are unable to recall the exact date, use the approximate year.
b. Surgeries and procedures. (If you do not remember the exact name, give a brief explanation.)
c. Complete as much history as you can remember and feel free to include all pertinent information that will be helpful during an emergency or medical treatment.
d. State if there is a particular medical condition that needs to be considered for future reference. Something that occurred even years prior could have an impact on a situation that is occurring today, and the medical team will need to know in order to better assist you with a diagnosis and recovery.
e. Make copies of the summary and keep a current master for your files.

1
Alerts and Concerns Log

It is important to list any medical, physical, or emotional areas of concern that requires attention. It will assist the caregiver of a medical condition that needs to be monitored and to also document when it occurs on the Medical Occurrence Form and the Chart Notes, as well as to notify the primary caregiver and possibly the physician.

This can be used when there is an emergency situation. Take a copy with you when you see a medical professional and give to the emergency team. This can help assist to better establish the cause of a medical situation quicker or to eliminate a possible procedure, especially in an emergency.

Be sure to keep the information up to date as situations arise.

Alerts and Concerns Log

It is important to list any medical, physical, or emotional areas of concern that requires attention.

Maintain a log for easy recall and review.

	Date	Condition	Concern
1.			
2.			
3.			
4.			
5.			
6.			
7.			
8.			
9.			
10.			
11.			
12.			
13.			
14.			
15.			
16.			
17.			
18.			
19.			
20.			

2
Allergy List

It is important for you to keep this up to date and include all allergies, especially if there are any that are life threatening. State what the medical condition is as well as any remedy instructions, medications to administer immediately, what to look for, and if an ambulance is needed. It is recommended to keep a list in the wallet for easy access.

- Foods
- Medication
- Herbal supplements
- Environmental, etc.

Food Allergy Card

Have a Food Allergy Card to show to the restaurant server who can show it to the manager and the cooks of any food allergies so they can help ensure your safety and for you to have a nice experience in the restaurant. We have them available upon request, or you can easily obtain a card in business card format from your local office supply store and print in your language and I recommend on using the back for another commonly used language in your area, for example, one side in English and the other in Spanish. Then you can have it laminated at your local your local business office center such as Kinkos, Staples, etc.

This has been a lifesaver for me as there have been many times when upon inquiry the server would think they do not use an allergy product in their restaurant and later when the card is shown to the chef or the manager, they would find out that it is the product that was actually used. There should be careful consideration or directions for a type of menu item so that it is safe to eat as well as in the kitchen to ensure that there is no cross contamination of the food preparation area with the kitchen tools used or the need to alter the recipe. When you are in a banquet setting, give your card to the hostess so they can have the banquet manager check for you. Do not be fooled that because it is an exclusive setting or high-quality facility, they always use top-end products and a preservative is not used if this is your allergy. It is to SAVE YOUR LIFE and to enjoy your time with your family and friends or just a time of solitude. Better safe than sorry or having to go to a hospital.

Example: You can state whatever you are comfortable with, but remember, this is to help keep you safe and possibly save your life depending on the allergy reaction. It is important to have your name included as either the manager or chef may want to meet you to discuss food options.

MY NAME (for the Manager to find you) **FOOD ALLERGIES**

Life Threatening *(examples of what to state)*

- **Dairy, gluten,**
- **Nuts, shellfish, etc.**

Additional Food Sensitivities:

- **List any foods here individually.**

On the back, you could repeat this in Spanish. If you do not know how to spell a word, you can ask someone who speaks the language, or in your grocery store, you could look for food labels on items where they are sometimes in English and Spanish so you can have a reference. Remember, depending on the country, the food item could be spelled differently so you may need to be alert for this.

Allergy List

❑ Medication ❖ ❑ Food ❖ ❑ Other

Keep Each Category on a Separate Page

	DATE	CAUSE OF ALLERGY State medication or food	REACTION Explain symptoms i.e., rash, anaphylaxis, etc.	REMEDY Counteractive action, i.e., specific medication
1.				
2.				
3.				
4.				
5.				
6.				
7.				
8.				
9.				
10.				
11.				
12.				
13.				
14.				
15.				
16.				
17.				
18.				
19.				
20.				

3
Caregiver

This area is meant for assisting the individual who will require a caregiver to assist with daily home care and the primary caregiver who is seeking assistance. Each area provides information from how to hire a caregiver, an interview sheet, and instructions once you have hired a caregiver or service.

Caregiver Agreement

This will provide a clear understanding of a written agreement with your caregiver. Make the appropriate changes.

Caregiver Daily Checklist

This is important to help establish what is needed for daily care. Many funding sources and social service programs qualify their services by the time and task needed for the individual's needs. Different tasks performed by a caregiver may appear simple and commonsense, but to a person being considered to assist with caregiving, it may not be a task normally done as each individual requires different considerations to maintain a continuity of health and care. This sample is meant to assist you in considering areas that you will want a caregiver to do. You may want a caregiver to use it daily; therefore, be sure to make copies so they can document that they have done each task as requested.

* Be sure to customize for the individual's needs.

* Also keep an updated copy in the Personal Care and Caregiver Handbooks.

Caregiver Employment Application

This is to be completed by the applicant. This will help during the interview to better understand the individual you are hiring.

Caregiver Guidelines

This provides the caregiver guidelines or expectations. Be sure to customize it to ensure clarity of understanding between you and the caregiver of their responsibilities and expectations.

Caregiver Hire Guidelines

I have supplied you with several forms that will give you example guidelines to put in your binder. It will be important for you to customize each area to ensure that your needs are met by adding pertinent information as this is <u>your</u> personalized handbook.

Caregiver Interview Checklist

This checklist provides you with guidelines when setting up for an interview.

Caregiver Interview Evaluation

The following is for YOUR REFERENCE ONLY. Areas are in general topics for reminders. Add additional specific topics and information that fit your needs. This helps in the applicant elimination process when you have interviewed several applicants. Many of the questions during an interview can reflect a gut feeling about someone. Once you become more familiar with the person and with the background check, you will be able to make a more informed hiring decision. You may want to get a picture to add to your file to help remind you of what the applicant looked like; you can use your cell phone in doing this.

Caregiver Interview Guidelines

The Caregiver Interview Guidelines offers a packet of information and assistance as part of the *Personal Care Handbook*, designed to provide some tools when you need to hire a new caregiver for your loved one or yourself.

Caregiver Interview Questionnaire

This is to be completed by the applicant so you can see if they meet your needs.

Caregiver Job Description

This is a sample to assist you. You can use some of it and add information or create your own; the choice is yours as this is meant as an example, and your specific needs must be stated to ensure that the applicant understands what is requested of their service.

Caregiver Agreement

This will provide a clear understanding of a written agreement with your caregiver. Make the appropriate changes.

DATE______________________

Employee ___________________________________ SS No. _______________________

Address ____________________________________ City _________________________

Zip __________________________ Driver's License No. _________________________

Phone __________________________ Other ___________________________________

In case of emergency: Name ______________________ Relationship _________________

Phone _________________ Or ______________________________

("I" in this document reflects the employee.)

1. I agree to work and perform the duties described on the job description and the daily program schedules discussed, as well as any other duties applicable.
2. I accept the salary of $________per hour and agree to work________hours daily.

   ❑ Monday ❑ Tuesday ❑ Wednesday ❑ Thursday ❑ Friday ❑ Saturday ❑ Sunday ❑ Holidays
3. I have a medical or physical restriction(s). ❑ YES ❑ NO

   It will create a problem or limitation to fulfill my daily duties. ❑ YES ❑ NO

   Please explain briefly.

   ____

   ____

   ____
4. I will not expect pay for any nonworking days to include sick days, holidays, personal days.
5. I understand that I will receive a schedule and sufficient notice not less than twenty-four (24) hours if I will not be needed unless an emergency or medical situation has occurred.
6. I have answered all the questions in the interview with accuracy and honesty.
7. I do not expect to receive medical insurance.
8. I understand I will be responsible for any tax reporting necessary.
9. I understand I will be paid by ❑ Personal or a ❑ Service____________________________

❑ Other____

ACCEPTED: ______________________________________ DATE____________
Employee

______________________________________ DATE____________
❑ Primary caregiver or ❑ Individual requiring the caregiver

Caregiver Daily Checklist

This is important to help establish what is needed for daily care. Many funding sources and social service programs qualify their services by the time and task needed for the individual's needs. Different tasks performed by a caregiver may appear simple and commonsense, but to a person being considered to assist with caregiving, it may not be a task normally done as each individual requires different considerations to maintain a continuity of health and care. This sample is meant to assist you to consider areas that you will want a caregiver to do. You may want a caregiver to use it daily; therefore, be sure to make copies so they can document that they have done each task as requested.

Be sure to customize for the individual's needs.
Also, keep an updated copy in the Personal Care and Caregiver Handbooks.

Name____Date__________________

It is important to offer assistance when applicable.
Please check each area after you have completed the task.

________TRANSPORT SERVICE to appointments if needed. Check the schedule for future appointments; some transport services require 24–48 hours' prior notification.

- Be sure to make the necessary transportation arrangements for all appointments.
- If you use a transport service, they will need *name, address, phone, appointment time.*
- See the Community Transport section for more instructions.

I. Shower, Personal Grooming Skills. Be sure to use gloves and ask what assistance is needed.

________ 1. Leave alone if requested. Stay close and within earshot, however, in the event you are needed.

________ 2. Transferring to shower or tub?

- If using a shower chair, assist with legs and feet protection and placement.
- Placing feet on a stool in the shower helps with stability and preventing hot water burns.

________ 3. Turn on water and check water temperature.

Legs and feet burns can occur from water being too hot.

________ 4. Assist to wash any areas difficult to reach as needed.

________ 5. Shower complete, check to ensure the water is turned off.

________ 6. Check frequently for decubitus sores.

________ a. After the shower is an easy time to do a quick visual body check for skin breakdowns, such as an open sore, redness, skin discoloration on the back area, buttock, elbows, legs, feet, and toes.

________ b. Clean and dry between the toes. Mention if the toenails need trimming or you notice a sore or any other condition that may need attention.

________ 7. Continue to ask if any assistance is needed.

________ 8. Leave alone to complete grooming skills if requested, staying close and within earshot in the event you are needed.

________ 9. Caregiver needs to do a visual check, remind, and/or assist in the following:

   a. Skin check
   b. Teeth cleaning
   c. Ears cleaning
   d. Application of deodorant
   e. Application of cologne, perfume
   f. Fingernails trimming, if applicable
   g. Shaving

Very Important: Ensure that briefs and pants are pulled up correctly so that it minimizes any bulk pressure against the skin when sitting. This can be a cause for a decubitus and needs to be monitored for correct placement of undergarment and pants.

________ 10. **Mention if you observe an odor. Locate source.**

   a. Urine: If there is a strong odor or discoloration, it could mean the possibility of a urinary tract infection (UTI). Contact the primary caregiver and/or the doctor on file.
   b. Incontinence: The individual may need a change, shower or bath.
   c. Sore: Needs immediate attention and to notify the primary caregiver and/or the doctor.
   d. Other____

________ 11. Notify primary caregiver of any **supplies** needed.

II. Preparation for Day. Use gloves as needed.

________ 1. Make bed. Check sheets and change if applicable. Put dirty sheets in the laundry room.

________ 2. Clean and straighten up bedroom. Vacuum and dust.

________ 3. Check the daily schedule of activities and pack the travel bag or backpack with appropriately needed supplies when leaving the home for any period of time.

________4. Assist with **daily medications** and what medications may need to be taken while on an outing.

- See Personal Bag Organization.
- If a prescription refill is needed, notify primary caregiver and/or individual.
- See Medication Daily Schedule and Chart.

________5. Prepare and assist with BREAKFAST and LUNCH.

________6. Prepare and assist with DINNER when needed. If leaving the food for later, cover and place in refrigerator.

________7. **Reminders.** Observe the individual and assist to prevent falls and regarding the following:

________ a. Intake of medications.

________ b. Monitoring of the Daily Vitals Checklist and Chart.

________ c. Charting the fluid intake if needed.

________ d. Using the Chart Notes section charting daily regarding the day's events, care, and any occurrence such as a fall or any other situation, especially noting any problems or concerns, to include grocery or supplies that will be needed.

________ e. Periodic weight shifting when sitting for long periods of time to help prevent decubitus ulcers. The physician or therapists may recommend the frequency.

________ f. Observance and assisting with incontinence care if applicable. If you smell or notice soiled clothing a change is needed.

________ g. Assist in the daily schedule of appointments and activities

________ h. Preparing for appointments and activities that will require assistance.

________ i. If transportation is needed contact a service and providing the information needed. (See the Community Transport section for more instructions.)

________8. **Cushion.** Use a waterproof pad to prevent from being soiled if applicable.

________ a. If used with a seating device, wheelchair, etc., check the following:

1. Is the cushion or cover soiled or smelly?
2. Do not wash the cushion in a washing machine as it will deteriorate the foam material unless otherwise directed.
3. Wash only the removable cover.
4. Follow the Equipment Maintenance section to know what you need to do.

________ b. Depending on its type, a cushion may require specific care. The individual or the primary caregiver will direct you or review the Equipment Maintenance section for more information.

________ c. For back cushion, check if in proper placement, if applicable.

________ d. Furniture cushion may need a waterproof pad.

________ 9. **Wheelchair**. Check if a repair is needed. Contact the primary caregiver.

________ a. If tire air pressure is low, assist with pumping tires or take to nearest bike shop.

________ b. Check if brakes and all parts are working correctly—that is, foot rest, arm rest, seat belts, etc.

________ c. Power chair batteries will need to be charged daily and checked periodically.

________ 10. **Housekeeping: Bedroom, Bathroom, Kitchen, General Living Areas.**

________ a. In the bathroom, completely clean the shower, bathtub, toilet, sinks, and floor daily.

________ b. With laundry, wash, dry, fold, and put away all laundry. Follow the instructions provided regarding the type of soap to use and all laundry products, as well as drying instructions.

- Be sure to notify the individual or primary caregiver when laundry products need to be purchased.

________ c. Clean kitchen. Wash, dry, and put away the dishes, leaving the kitchen neat and in order.

________ d. Vacuum and mop floors as needed.

________ e. Dust the surface areas as directed and needed.

________ f. Water plants as directed and needed.

________ g. Make a list of any groceries, cleaning and laundry items needed from the store.

III. Other. Please list all that you want to be handled.

1. ______ (Prompt to drink to keep hydrated, e.g.)
2. ______ (Frequency in changing incontinence care, e.g.)
3. ______ ________________________________
4. ______ ________________________________
5. ______ ________________________________
6. ______ ________________________________
7. ______ ________________________________
8. ______ ________________________________
9. ______ ________________________________
10. ______ ________________________________

Caregiver Employment Application

Please complete and return.

Personal Information Date____________________

Name____Social Security No.__________

Address____

City______________________________________State__________Zip__________

Phone_____________________________________Cell____________________

E-mail____

Employment Desired

Position____________________Date you can start____________________

Salary Desired ____

Are you employed? ❑ Yes ❑ No ______________________________________

Education History

High School______________________________________Year graduated__________

College or trade school_____________________________Year graduated__________

Field of interest ❑ Nursing ____________________________❑ LVN ❑ NA ❑ OT ❑ PT

License Type /Specialty

❑ Other ____

Graduation/Certification____

General Information

Special training____

____

____

Prior Employment **Okay to contact for reference**____________

1. Name ____Phone______________

Date started__________________________Ended____________________

Reason for leaving____

Please explain briefly job duties____________________________________

____

2. Name ______________________________ Phone ______________

Date started ______________________ Ended ______________

Reason for leaving ______________________________________

Please explain briefly job duties ________________________

____

Caregiver Guidelines

This provides the caregiver guidelines of expectations. You can customize it to ensure clarity. A caregiver professional should add value to the daily life of the individual. Consider your position as an important aspect for the safety of the person you care for as it is an honor to care for another person.

Remember, you are *not babysitting* but assisting an individual who has special needs with their daily care.

Ways to protect yourself:

- Take a notepad with you when you go to work to ensure you have paper to write down all information needed. Remember to leave it, as you do not need to take it with you since it is personal information. Ask your client where you can leave your notes for future reference.
- Documenting your work will assist you to keep the family informed.
- Accurate documentation of your participation in their daily care adds value to your skills, giving you the opportunity to show the individual and the family you care for their health and safety.
- Should a situation arise, you will know through your documentation you did what was needed.
- Always state any area of care that makes you uncomfortable immediately. This will protect you and allows the individual or primary caregiver to make any necessary changes.

Ask specific information for the following:

1. Individual's name and pertinent information.
    a. What is the medical condition or disability, that is, cognitive issues, stroke victim, dementia, other?
    b. Do you distribute medications, and what is the frequency?
    c. Are there any mobility limitations? Are there any specific instructions?
        i. Do they need assistance in walking, for example, with a cane, walker, etc.?
        ii. Do they need assistance in transfers from a bed, chair, commodes, etc.?
        iii. In what other areas does the individual needs to be kept safe or monitored?
    d. Are there any specific medical concerns that you need to monitor or watch for?
    e. If you need to assist with a medical procedure, what do you do, that is, vitals, insulin monitoring, shots, other?

2. Address and cross street (In the event of an emergency—*we get nervous and having this information is important.*)
3. House phone number
4. Contact information of primary caregiver
5. If an emergency occurs, who do you contact?
6. Are there any pets in the home, and do you have any responsibility to them? If you are uncomfortable with this, please state your concerns immediately.
7. What are your duties and responsibilities?
    a. Food preparation
        i. Are there any restrictions or allergies?
        ii. Are there any prepared meals to warm?
        iii. If you are asked to cook, are there any meal suggestions?
    b. Liquid intake: in drinking, do you need to prompt to drink?
    c. Hygiene care: what is involved, how much do you need to do?
        i. Do you assist with showers/baths? Personal grooming? Be sure to find out explicitly in this area so it is not uncomfortable for you or the individual.
        ii. This is time to check if there are any open sores or red pressure marks.
        iii. Change the briefs (diaper) to ensure they are properly clean.
    d. Changing the bed linen and towels
    e. Washing laundry, drying, folding, and where to put them in the appropriate cupboard or shelf. As well what laundry products do they want to be used for the different type of washing loads and drying instructions.
    f. How do you use the various appliances such as the washing machine and dryer?
    g. Vacuum the bedroom and living area?
    h. Dusting?
    i. Cleaning bathroom?
    j. Taking garbage out and the location of the outside garbage container?
    k. Any other chores requested?
8. Medical situation has occurred or you notice a problem, what do you do?
    a. Be sure you give your report to the primary caregiver.
    b. Document what happened.
        i. Who do you contact, and where are the phone numbers?
        ii. Be sure to include in your documentation who you reported the situation to and include the time and date.
        iii. Sign your name, as this will be needed for future reference.
    c. If 911 is called, is the following information available?
        i. A specific medical facility to go to

ii. Doctor's name and phone number
iii. Insurance information
iv. All medical card numbers and their location, to include state/federal agency qualifying programs; e.g. Medi-Cal for California
v. Medical history summary
vi. Medication list or the medication in their Rx containers
vii. All food and medication allergies
viii. Is there a personal medical history journal to document what has occurred when going to the hospital or medical appointment?

d. Have you documented accurately what you did to assist before and after the emergency team arrived?

BE SURE TO ASK IF THERE IS ANYTHING YOU SHOULD BE AWARE OF!

Caregiver Hire Guidelines

The supplied forms within each area give you example guidelines to put in your binder. It will be important for you to customize each area to ensure your needs are met by adding pertinent information as this is your personalized handbook.

1. **Caregiver interview checklist**. This will provide guidelines when setting up for an interview.
   a. For the initial interview meeting, **DO NOT MEET AT HOME**, meet at a fast food, coffee shop, or some other neutral location.
   b. Review the questions and add important areas that you want to ensure are covered.
   c. You may want to get a picture of the person to add to your file, you can use your cell phone to help remind you of what the applicant looked like.
   d. **DO NOT HIRE UNTIL** you have a personal interview and have gone through all the background and reference checks.
   e. If the person does not sound like they will work out, say so and thank them for the call or interview.
   f. You may really like the person, but they may be apprehensive about the care. Do not try to make the person do anything they are not comfortable doing. You have the option to limit the chores they will do, but remember, someone will have to do it!
   g. Be sure to add a separate sheet or notebook with additional questions you may have.

2. **Caregiver job description**
   a. Requires your individualized comments.
   b. Have this with you when you interview and show the person you are interviewing so they can see what is expected of their service.

3. **Caregiver employment application and questionnaire**
   a. Because you will require specific care needs, you may want to modify this form.
   b. This needs to be completed by the prospective caregiver. Have them fill it in prior to interviewing or visiting with them so you can reference it when talking to them.

4. **Caregiver guidelines**. This should be given to the prospective caregiver to provide guidelines for questions and expectations.

5. **<u>Caregiver daily checklist</u>**. Be sure to make the appropriate changes.
   a. Make a <u>detailed list</u> of your expectations of care to ensure that all needs are met.
   b. Every time you do even a simple task, add it to your list; that is, get drinks, simple reminders, etc.
   c. The caregiver is hired to assist the individual with their care and assistance with their needs in the home, <u>not</u> the entire household chores unless you make other arrangements.
   d. Caregiver household chores list: clean the bathroom and kitchen daily, laundry, vacuum, mop, dust, cooking, shopping, etc., <u>not</u> babysitting, watching TV, or reading.
   e. You <u>may</u> want to hire another person to clean the home weekly or biweekly depending on your needs. The caregiver could do the surface cleaning and another person or service to handle the more intense cleaning.

6. **<u>Caregiver interview evaluation</u>**
   a. This is for your reference only and best for your records as it is not intended to be shared with the applicant.
   b. Areas are in general topics for reminders.
   c. Add additional specific topics and information that fit your needs.
   d. The responses to the questions during an interview can give you a gut feeling about someone. Once you become more familiar with the person and with the background check, you will be able to make a more informed decision regarding hiring.
   e. This helps in the elimination applicant process when you have interviewed several applicants.

<u>Important Safeguards to Consider</u>

<u>Insurance.</u> When hiring a caregiver be sure to contact your personal insurance agent to ensure you are protected in the event of a claim regarding the following, and ask the type of coverage it offers.

a. It is recommended to add a workers' compensation insurance policy to your homeowners policy. The premium is generally extremely low, and it gives you important protection. If you are working with a health provider service they may have a policy so be sure to request a copy or Certificate of Insurance so you know you are protected. Do not assume, because they have a business, that they have the appropriate insurance that protects the employee and you, so always ask.
b. Mention to your personal automobile agent that the hired caregiver may use your vehicle for errands to ensure you have the appropriate coverage; or, the hired caregiver may use their personal vehicle and you want to insure if they are driving your loved one to

appointments, errands, or anything that they have the appropriate insurance coverage. Ask for an Insurance Certificate, and to be sure the coverage is appropriate you can have your personal agent review it.

Discrimination. Be careful not to discriminate due to religion, race, or sex. Be open to the individual who has the appropriate experience to handle your needs safely. However, it is okay to state up front that the person who requires the care may be more comfortable with a specific person, such as a male or a female.

a. A small-structured female may not be able to handle an adult male when transferring or when handling incontinence issues.
b. A female may be very uncomfortable with a male caregiver.

State and local required documents. Contact the following local offices for the required documents when hiring an employee.

a. Labor Commissioner Office
b. Employment Development Department

Be sure to ask if there are other offices to locate and obtain the contact information as well as any areas and helpful suggestions to be considered.

Health service provider. This is an important service as they are experienced and handle all the background checks needed and more. There is an additional charge but well worth the additional comfort of knowing you have done your best when hiring someone to care for your loved one and who is coming into your home.

a. Fingerprinting.
b. Credit report checks.
c. Felony or misdemeanors.
d. Motor vehicle records (important if they are going to drive for you).
e. Drug testing.
f. Reference checks.
g. Ask what other services are offered.

Payroll. This can get difficult with the payroll taxes if you are personally handling and not using a health service provider. If personally handling, you may want to contact a payroll service to assist you as you are required to pay and file the state and federal taxes and appropriate reporting.

Caregiver personnel file. Keep a copy of all the hiring and payroll information for each caregiver in their individual personnel file.

Appliance and equipment

a. Have instructions for each household appliance used, such as the washing machine (how to separate clothes, types of laundry products used, etc.); clothes dryers (i.e., clean lint filter); coffee maker; and others.
b. If there is a particular equipment they need to check or use, it will be important to have instructions. You can use the Equipment Maintenance section to assist you.

Home protection/security

a. Put a lock on any door the caregiver will not need to enter.
b. Protect all valuables, medications, and place in a secured location that will not be accessible.
c. Contact a local security monitoring service for options and suggestions, and you may want to add cameras. Using these services provides you to go online via your computer and on cell phones to view what is occurring while you are away.
d. You can get a nanny cam type of camera available online to help monitor what the caregiver is doing when you are not present.
e. Be sure to keep the bills, all receipts, and any personal information in a protected location to help prevent identity theft.

Caregiver Interview Checklist

This checklist provides you with guidelines when setting up for an interview.

Name____Date__________

Phone ❑ Cell________________❑ Home_______________❑ Other____________

E-mail____

1. Discuss basic chores before meeting. If still interested, then arrange for a meeting.
2. Set up: Date_____________ Time________Location___________________
3. Job Description. Have a copy for the prospective caregiver to review and return.
4. Employment Application. Have the interviewee complete and review each area with them during the interview.
   ☑ Check the following: (Gives you an idea of their schedule availability.)
5. Attending College________________________________
   - ❑ Full time ❑ Part time
   - ❑ Availability Days _________ Hours ________________
   - ❑ Units________Major_________________________
6. Employed Where ____
   - ❑ Full time ❑ Part time
   - ❑ Availability Days________________Hours__________
   - ❑ Can I contact them______If yes, ask for the supervisor name and phone.

   ____
7. Caregiver Questionnaire. For you to use to ask questions for the interview.
8. Caregiver Daily Checklist. Discuss duties explicitly.
9. Show Personal Caregiver Handbook with the different sections.
   a. Explain Medical History Summary to understand the medical condition.
   b. Emergencies or Medical Attention**. WHAT TO LOOK FOR AND WHOM TO CONTACT**
   c. Equipment. Be sure to mention any equipment and supplies used. (See the Equipment Maintenance section.)
10. Ask if he/she is interested in the job. This is also a time for you to decide if you want to hire this person.
11. Inform the person if you work with a health service provider and that they will handle all background, credit, fingerprinting, and reference checks. Ask if this is agreeable; if not, it can be a clue not to hire.
12. Discuss when you will get back to them regarding the hiring decision, time and date______

13. Notify the health service provider with the name and phone number of the prospective caregiver to begin the background, drug, and credit check.
14. Once you have made a decision to hire, give the prospective caregiver the number to the health service provider you have selected to begin the process.
15. Salary $_______. Have a range. Start low, but it must be at least minimum wage. However, it is best to have it slightly higher than minimum wage depending on what would be required.
16. Be sure if you will be using a funding source to cover the salary, explain what they will need to do to register with the service provider needed to maintain a continuity of health. Check with your local university or medical teaching centers to see if they can offer the medical support you may need. As well, you will need to see what funding programs can be helpful in providing assistance.

    Some of the support and funding programs require information even as far back as infancy for acceptance into their program when working as an adult at any age. Ms. Lopez has been witness to a situation where a family member with medical issues that require daily monitoring and assistance is in his late sixties and has been under the care of his mother for his entire life. The mother is getting on with age, and the siblings are trying to get program funding and services to help their brother. Because he was not in the various programs available in his earlier years, they must supply information back to his childhood, which has been very difficult to locate. This caused problems in being accepted into various programs, as well as to understand all that is needed to care for their brother. If there had been a file or some type of information in the family files, it would have been easier, especially in a time they are also dealing with the issues of the parent.

    - Ensure you understand the hourly wages provided by the service provider and the prospective employee accepts the wages.
    - You will have an option to add another source or personal funds to provide a higher wage.
    - It will be important to discuss the various salary funding options and ask if they accept.
17. Hours. List days and times required.
18. Employment duration. Length of time available for employment_________________
19. Any existing medical conditions with limitations that would prevent doing what is required? (i.e., back problems, disability, walking or lifting limitations, etc.). You can decide if this person is appropriate for your needs if a disability will prevent them from fulfilling what is needed.

Use this section to add any questions you may have.

________ 20. ____

________ 21. ____

________ 22. ____

________ 23. ____

________ 24. ____

________ 25. ____

________ 26. ____

________ 27. ____

________ 28. ____

________ 29. ____

________ 30. ____

________ 31. ____

________ 32. ____

________ 33. ____

________ 34. ____

________ 35. ____

________ 36. ____

________ 37. ____

________ 38. ____

________ 39. ____

________ 40. ____

Caregiver Interview Evaluation

A. The following is for YOUR REFERENCE ONLY. Areas are in general topics for reminders. Add additional specific topics and information that fit your needs.
B. This helps in the applicant elimination process when you have interviewed several applicants.
C. Many of the questions during an interview can reflect a gut feeling about someone.
D. Once you become more familiar with the person and with the background check, you will be able to make a more informed hiring decision.
E. You may want to get a picture to add to your file to help remind you of what the applicant looked like; you can use your cell phone for this.

NAME____**Date**__________

<u>Health Service Provider.</u> Contact for background checks and start date of employment

Name____
Contact__________________________________Phone__________
Address____
E-mail____

______1. **<u>Prospective Caregiver APPEARS.</u>** You can review their personal appearance and vehicle to see if it is kept clean and neat. Watch for any other clue that will help you to see how they will care for your needs.

❑ YES ❑ NO a. Dependable.
❑ YES ❑ NO b. Honest.
❑ YES ❑ NO c. Able to work independently.
❑ YES ❑ NO d. Social lifestyles compatible.
❑ YES ❑ NO e. Would you be comfortable with this person in your home when you are not present?
❑ YES ❑ NO f. Does he/she appear neat?

______2. **<u>Personality</u>**

❑ YES ❑ NO a. Friendly.
❑ YES ❑ NO b. Appears to get along with others.
❑ YES ❑ NO c. Enjoys working with families with special needs.

_______3. **Hours**

❑ YES ❑ NO a. Willing to work flexible hours, different shifts. ❑ AM ❑ Afternoon ❑ PM ❑ Evenings

❑ YES ❑ NO b. Attends college.

❑ YES ❑ NO If yes, are the hours flexible enough to accommodate both schedules?

❑ YES ❑ NO c. Do they have another job?

❑ YES ❑ NO If yes, are the hours flexible enough to accommodate both schedules?

❑ YES ❑ NO d. Flexible. Able to assist with your time management as needed and willing to adjust to change regarding working hours.

_______4. **Duties**

❑ YES ❑ NO a. Willing to do cleaning, cooking, and domestic chores, either assigned or as needed?

i. Reviewed the Job Description.

ii. Reviewed the Caregivers Daily Checklist that includes household chores of what will be expected.

❑ YES ❑ NO b. Accepts the personal care duties and responsibilities; i.e., issues of bowel, bladder, vomiting, etc. If not, in what areas?____

_______5. **Medical Knowledge**

❑ YES ❑ NO a. Has had medical training? If yes, explain.______________________________

❑ YES ❑ NO b. Licensed? If yes, explain.____

❑ YES ❑ NO c. Has the basic knowledge of what to do in an emergency.

❑ YES ❑ NO d. CPR First Aid Certified?

❑ YES ❑ NO If no, willing to take a class? *Note*: Offered through the American Red Cross or online.

_______6. **References**. *Note*: If the reference is family or a friend, you will only receive positive comments.

❑ YES ❑ NO a. Willing to work with a health service provider who will do a complete background check, fingerprinting, and drug testing that will include all references verified.

❑ YES ❑ NO b. Reports from health service provider are in good standing. If not, you can ask the person what occurred; and if they explain, then you have the opportunity to make the final decision to hire.

_______7. **Drives**

❑ YES ❑ NO a. Have the health service provider check the motor vehicle report (MVR).

❑ YES ❑ NO b. Do they have a vehicle available to handle errands and appointments, such as going to the pharmacy, taking a specimen to a laboratory, going to the grocery store or to another location?

❑ YES ❑ NO c. If yes, are they willing to use their vehicle?

❑ YES ❑ NO d. Proof of automobile insurance limits? Ask for a copy of their insurance declaration page to see what type of coverage limits they have.
Note: Add to your personal insurance the nonowned vehicle coverage to ensure that if they are doing errands, you are covered under your auto policy. Check with your insurance agent to ensure that you have the insurance protection.

❑ YES ❑ NO e. Travel. If willing to accompany on a trip for any period of time.
Note: This would be used on an individual basis or until some time in the future as an option, once you have decided if you can trust this individual.

_______8. **Salary**

❑ YES ❑ NO a. Has accepted the salary range offered $________per hour. It is best to have an hourly rate.

❑ YES ❑ NO b. Willing to accept payment from other funding agencies?

_______9. **Medical Conditions**. You can ask your service provider if they can ask the personal health questions. A health service provider can ask some of the delicate questions.

❑ YES ❑ NO a. Do they have any medical condition that would limit them from doing what is requested? You do have the right to ask this question.
Discuss this area with your health service provider to ensure they give you the legal guidelines to follow in your state or local area or they can ask the questions and report the responses to you. Make an additional list to ensure that your needs are met.

Here are a few areas to consider:

❑ YES ❑ NO a. Lifting. Any weight restrictions?
If yes, get an explanation.

❑ YES ❑ NO b. Mobility issues?
What type of mobility issues?

❑ YES ❑ NO c. Disabled?
What is the disability?

❑ YES ❑ NO d. Hepatitis positive?

❑ If not, have they had their immunizations?

❑ If yes, what precautions are needed for the individual?

❑ YES ❑ NO e. TB tests. You want to be sure they have a current and negative result.

❑ YES ❑ NO f. HIV test?

❑ If positive, what precautions are needed for the client?

❑ YES ❑ NO g. Are they diabetic, is there anything that would limit them or require ensuring they are insulin balanced?

_______10. **Pets.** Be sure to discuss all types of animals in the home.

❑ YES ❑ NO a. Will they work with the pets in the home?

❑ YES ❑ NO b. Are there any concerns regarding the pets? Ask to explain.________________

____

_______11. **Hired. BE SURE TO WAIT UNTIL ALL THE BACKGROUND REPORTS HAVE RETURNED.**

❑ YES ❑ NO a. Date contacted regarding the decision to hire or not:

❑ YES ❑ NO b. When available to start: Date________________Day______________

Hours ❑ Daily______❑ Weekly

Schedule: ❑ Sunday ❑ Monday ❑ Tuesday ❑ Wednesday ❑ Thursday ❑ Friday ❑ Saturday

Times:__________ __________ __________ __________ __________ __________

Note____

Caregiver Interview Guidelines

The Caregiver Interview Guidelines offers a packet of information and assistance as part of the *Personal Care Handbook* designed to provide some tools when you need to hire a new caregiver for your loved one or yourself.

Here are some suggestions to handle the process:

1. When hiring the person yourself, it is important to take the appropriate safeguards as stated below.
   a. Be sure to obtain workers' compensation insurance. Contact your insurance agent who may be able to add it to your current policy for a minimal charge. Some policies require a separate policy check into it to see the advantages for you, and if the cost is very minimal annually, it could be a safeguard against the person submitting a claim.
2. Hiring through a health service provider—highly recommended.
   a. Contact a local health service provider to arrange all the background, credit, fingerprinting checks, drug testing, and all additional report.
   b. Ask their advice.
   c. It is recommended to utilize this service for a minimum of ninety (90) days for the caregiver's probationary period. This will also give you added protection since they will be under the health service providers workers' compensation insurance.
   d. Generally, during this time you will be able to find out if the caregiver is the appropriate person to meet your needs; and if not, it can prevent a workers' compensation insurance claim.
   e. It allows you to release the employee quickly and the opportunity to allow the service provider to send someone who may be more qualified; thus, you would not experience a break in the care until you locate another full-time caregiver and start the process again.
   f. Using a health service provider will have an additional cost because they are paying the workers' compensation insurance, all the employee taxes, and it will include their fees.
      i. Be sure to inform them you have a binder with various customized forms the caregiver will be expected to complete daily even though they may have something.
      ii. It will give you protection to utilize their experience and advice.

iii. It also gives you time, ninety (90) days, to see if the person you hired is appropriate for your needs.

iv. Negotiate with the health service provider on their hourly salary under their contract. Remember that you must pay the minimum wage, and ask the length of time needed to be kept under their contract until you can have the person under your direct payroll. This would mean you would be completely responsible for the person's payroll, taxes, and workers' compensation insurance.

v. Generally, a caregiver does not expect health benefits, vacation or sick leave pay as this can be an option should you want to offer.

vi. You can start the person at a lower hourly wage and increase once they have completed their ninety (90) day probation and under your payroll versus the health service provider.

vii. You may want to consider a payroll service who will handle all the taxes and filings required.

It is recommended utilizing the Web to search for information to assist you. Here are a few references:

1. www.AARP.org. You may need to be creative in searching for some of your answers, but I have found they have good information that can be used for any age regarding caregivers and finding a facility to assist you with a loved one.
2. www.CareInHomes.com. They have a very informative interactive Web site.
3. Check the search engines with the topic on the type of disability, caregiver, home facilities, etc.

Caregiver Interview Questionnaire

Applicant (Please complete and return to the person you are interviewing with.)

DATE____________________

NAME____PHONE____________________

E-MAIL____CELL_____________________

❑ Male ❑ Female

Field of Interest: ❑ Nursing________________________________❑ LVN ❑ NA ❑ OT ❑ PT

License Type /Specialty

❑ Other____

1. How many years of education have you completed?_________________________
2. ❑ YES ❑ NO Are you new to the area? *Explain.*_____________________________
3. What types of work have you done and liked the best?________________________

   ____
4. ❑ YES ❑ NO Do you have previous experience working with a person with a disability? *Explain.*____
5. What are your feelings toward disabilities?_____________________________
6. How do you deal with boredom and stress?_____________________________
7. ❑ YES ❑ NO Will you be able to drive or accompany to appointments when needed?
8. ❑ YES ❑ NO Are you comfortable using your vehicle for errands and/or doctor appointments?

   ❑ YES ❑ NO Do you have car insurance?

   You will be requested to provide a copy of the declaration sheet from your auto policy that shows the coverage limits if you will be driving your car for errands and doctor appointments and a copy of your current motor vehicle record.
9. ❑ YES ❑ NO Do you have any physical or emotional limitations that would limit your job?

   If you are comfortable to explain further, please use the back side of this paper.
10. ❑ YES ❑ NO Are you comfortable with lifting and assisting with transfers.

    Explain any limitations.____
11. ❑ YES ❑ NO Can you work independently?
12. ❑ YES ❑ NO Do you mind working with nudity that goes along with personal care?

    Explain any limitations.____
13. ❑ YES ❑ NO Will you do laundry—wash, dry, fold, and put away?
14. ❑ YES ❑ NO Will you do food preparation and cooking?
15. ❑ YES ❑ NO Will you do household chores? Make bed, clean up bathroom, etc.?
16. ❑ YES ❑ NO Would you be willing to wear the caregiver attire (scrubs or other). *This is an optional personal preference if you want them not to wear their street clothes while at work.*

17. ❑ YES ❑ NO____
18. ❑ YES ❑ NO____
19. ❑ YES ❑ NO____
20. ❑ YES ❑ NO____

Caregiver Job Description

This is a sample to assist you. You can use some of it and add information or create your own, the choice is yours as this is meant as an example, and your specific needs must be stated to ensure the applicant understands what is requested of their service.

Date______________________

DISABILITY ____

CLIENT ❑ Male ❑ Female: ❑ Young ❑ Teenager ❑ 21+ older ❑ _________age if applicable, etc.

DUTIES. ***Be sure to personalize anything important for your individual needs.***

1. Review each section of your *Personal Care Handbook* or the *Personal Caregivers Handbook.*
2. Use the Caregiver Daily Checklist to review the daily chores.
    a. Assist with monitoring daily health concerns, guidance, and assistance as needed.
    b. Skin inspection for decubitus, fractures, sores, burns, etc.
    c. Assist with food preparation.
    d. Monitor medication intake and notify primary caregiver if a refill is needed.
    e. Take vitals as needed or required.
    f. When you notice an important medical condition, incident, or illness, notify primary caregiver immediately.
    g. Assist with transfers when applicable.
    h. Assist to reorder medical supplies, if applicable.
    i. Light housekeeping. Review Caregivers Daily Checklist.
        i. Assist with keeping bathroom and bedroom clean.
        ii. Make bed and change sheets when applicable.
        iii. Wash, fold, and put laundry away.
        iv. Complete the Caregivers Daily Checklist.
    j. Accompany to doctor appointments or trips (optional).

Provide a resume and a referral list of three (3) past employment references with phone numbers to contact that are not family or friends.

Contact Person (*Name)*_________________________________**Phone**_______________

HOURS HOURS NEEDED. *Hours may be flexible depending on daily needs.*

Weekly Total__________________

Morning__________________

Afternoon__________________

	Evening________________________
	Other *(explain)*____
DAYS NEEDED	❑ Monday ❑ Tuesday ❑ Wednesday ❑ Thursday ❑ Friday ❑ Saturday ❑ Sunday
PAY	$______________ ❑ Per Hour ❑ Weekly ❑ Monthly
TIME CARD	Maintain approved hours by ❑ primary caregiver, ❑ case manager or ❑ other____________
BENEFITS	❑ None ❑ Health ❑ Other *(explain)*__________________________________

4
Chart Notes

- Use this form to leave a note regarding an occurrence, medical concern, or as a daily update.
- This will alert the family, primary caregiver, or any other caregiver on a situation that has occurred or requires monitoring.
- This is important to be sure you have protected your client if a fall occurred or there was something out of the ordinary.
- It is IMPORTANT to notify by phone, unless you have been instructed otherwise, the primary caregiver and the physician if a situation occurs that will require any medical attention.

Chart Notes

Use this form to leave a note for the primary caregiver or individual regarding an occurrence, medical concern, or as a daily update.

Day________________ **Date**________________ **Time**________________

PERSON CHARTING ☐ Caregiver ☐ Nurse ☐ Family ☐ Other________________

NAME________________________________**TITLE**________________

TEMPERATURE________________ **BLOOD PRESSURE**________________

SKIN

☐ Good ☐ Discoloration________________________ ☐ Wound (Describe below.)

URINE

Color ☐ Clear ☐ Brown/Red (Bloody) ☐ Odor ☐ Other (Describe below.)

1. AREA OF CONCERN ☐ NONE ☐ Allergies ☐ Fractures ☐ Infection ☐ Other

____

____

Explain/comment ____

____

____

____

____

____

2. AREA OF CONCERN ☐ NONE ☐ Allergies ☐ Fractures ☐ Infection ☐ Other

____

____

Explain/comment ____

____

____

____

____

____

Signed ____________________________ Notified __________________

5
Community Transportation

Guidelines to assist with mobility instructions for any form of community transportation; bus, train, muni, rapid transit system, etc.

It is important to assist the individual with special needs to have the self-confidence so that they can be more mobile with your assistance. Getting a person out of their home environment can provide good self-esteem, the opportunity to be in more social gatherings if at the mall and moving around, to the doctor's visit, store, a church gathering, a movie, school, a time to meet a friend or family, or sports event. It offers a feeling of independence and strength.

There are several options available in an area. Some funding services offer taxi or community transit free passes, so be sure to inquire what is available in your area. Ask the distance any one service will provide and if there will be an additional charge.

It is recommended to travel with the individual at first until they are comfortable to be alone. If handling a public transit system, you may want to follow in your vehicle to ensure they get off at the designated destination for a few times until you and they are comfortable to handle it independently.

Be sure to instruct the individual to tell the driver what exit point they will need and to ask where to pick up the return transport vehicle or bus.

Note that some of the paratransit services may not be on your time frame for the pickup or delivery. They may come early or later. So be sure to ask how much time is needed to be ready prior to pickup and the location to meet, as well as the approximate time they may be delivered to their destination.

If taking any supplies, be sure to have them properly marked in the event they get left on the transport vehicle so the people can notify you they have the bag or item that was left.

Community Transportation

The following are guidelines when assisting an individual with mobility for any form of community transportation: bus, train, muni, rapid transit system, etc.

I. ROUTING: Instructions

1. Request local transit schedule - disabled access guide.
   a. Call a local transit service.
   b. Ask for their best route.
   c. Refer to the transportation guide that discusses the schedule, whom to call for information, emergencies, etc.
   d. A community transport service may pick up at the home, take to the destination, and pick up for the return trip.

2. Use index cards.
   a. Using a hole punch, put a hole in upper corner.
   b. Put ring or string through for more than one card.
   c. On each index card, write the following:______________________________
   (The following is an example however applicable to any type of transportation system.)

→ ***Side 1***

✓ **To**____________________________
✓ **From**__________________________
✓ **Destination**_____________________

✓ **Times of departure**________________
____
____

✓ **Bus number**_____________________
✓ **Location**_______________________
✓ **Departs / Leaves**_________________

✓ **Transfers: How many**__________
✓ **Bus number**_____________________
✓ **Location**_______________________
✓ **Departs / Leaves**_________________

✓ **Destination**______________________

✶ Be sure to ask the driver for assistance if needed and the location of the pickup area.

→ ***Side 2:*** On the back of index card, write the return information.

Use the same format as on the front side.

3. Keep information simple; use large writing.

II. BEFORE LEAVING checklist

1. Take the index card and check time frames.
   a. Call the transportation company for assistance:
      ✓Verify times, current line number (*such as bus number*), route, etc.
      ✓If a lift is required for a wheelchair or any type of assistance needed for individual needs, would they be available?
   b. Allow extra time to get to and from bus stop to the destination.
   c. Keep an ID card in travel pack that has the name, address, bus line needed, phone number, emergency information.
   d. Fill backpack for travel with supplies and extra clothing.
   e. Take bottle of water.
   f. Be sure any medications needed during the time away from home is packed.

III. AT BUS STOP

1. **Ramp Safety**
   a. Stay clear from the ramp while in motion.
   b. Wheelchair users generally back onto ramp.
   c. Wheelchair users put brakes on when on the ramp.
   d. Transport services, buses, etc., will not allow a wheelchair without a seat belt and properly working brakes.

2. **On Bus Locking System**
   a. Be sure the chair is secured to the locking system by the transport driver.
   b. Some transport systems also have a seat belt that goes around the wheelchair.
   c. Apply brakes on wheelchair.

3. **Upon Reaching Destination**
    a. Inform the driver of the destination when entering the bus.
    b. Brace for all stops.
    c. Inform the driver before reaching the stop.
    d. Okay to ask for help, directions, etc.
    e. Ask the driver where the pickup location is for the return trip.
    f. Check the cross streets needed to reach the return-bus location.

IV. CROSSWALK SAFETY

a. Use wheelchair ramps
b. Use pedestrian crosswalk buttons, if available
c. Carefully check for vehicle drivers not watching—**be alert!**

NOTE to travel independently:

a. It is strongly recommended that a caregiver travels with the individual a few times to be sure there is an understanding of the transportation routine.
b. When traveling independently, have someone follow in a car to ensure they know their route and get to their destination.

6
Emergency Contact Information

The individual or the primary caregiver needs to complete this information for quick access of important contact information in the event an emergency occurs.

Place a copy on a cabinet or refrigerator in the kitchen and any other location so it is easily visible and easily accessed.

Emergency Contact Information

Keep this in the caregiver binder and post in an area where it is easily accessible in the event there is an emergency.

Name ____________________

Address ____________________

Home Phone ____________________ Other ____________________

Nearest intersection ____________________

Medical Care Service Provider ____________________ Phone ____________________

In an Emergency ❑ Medical History Available ❑ Allergies ❑ Medication ❑ Foods ❑ _____

Call 911 and/or ❑ Primary Caregiver ____________________

Mobile Phone ____________________ Other ____________________

Doctor ____________________ Phone____________________

Hospital/Medical Facility ____________________

Medical Insurance Carrier ____________________ ID No. ____________________

Additional Contact:

Name ____________________

Relationship ____________________ Phone ____________________

Additional Important Contacts:

State if family, friend, or other ____________________

____

Information to provide the medical team, physician, emergency team, etc.

Take the following:

- ❑ ID and insurance cards (generally found in a wallet unless otherwise directed by primary caregiver)

- ❑ The *Personal Caregiver Handbook* ❑ *Personal Medical Journal* ❑ *Personal Medical Summary*
- ❑ Personal and medical supplies (a medical facility may not have the preferred supplies)
- ❑ All medication bottles and the Medication Daily Schedule

❑ The following individual sheets from the *Personal Caregiver Handbook*

- ❑ Current Daily Vitals Record-Keeping Log ❑ Medical Concerns Checklist ❑ Alerts and Concerns Log
- ❑ Allergy List
- ❑ ______________________________
- ❑ ______________________________

Additional Information ❑ Use the Community Transportation Instruction Section

<u>Transportation</u>

Service ______________________________ Taxi______________________________

____

7
Equipment Maintenance

It is important to have information on each equipment used, the vendor's contact number if a repair is necessary, and where specific equipment or supplies can be ordered.

Keeping the information in an area that is simple to access along with the care instructions will enable the caregiver to know how to care and whom to contact for repairs or reorder of specific supplies for each piece of equipment that is used.

The attached information will also give you pertinent information on general equipment as to what to consider when purchasing an item, how to use, care for, and precautions for any equipment that is utilized. It will be important to customize it for your needs. There may be areas that you specifically need to have considered or to add a section when reordering or placing an order on an item.

Separating each equipment provides an easy way to find them. Be sure to fill in sections of this form for you to customize to meet your needs.

Equipment Maintenance

Complete this form customizing it to meet your needs.

Be sure to add all equipment and the specific needs for its care. Be sure to add additional pages with your information on any equipment you may have that is not included.

CONTACT 1. Primary caregiver ❑ See list____________________ Phone____________________
2. Mobility service provider____________________ Phone____________________

This section includes information on a variety of equipment used and areas to consider regarding the purpose of the equipment, initial ordering, and more on the following:

- I. Wheelchair
- II. Cushions, seating and back
- III. Shower chair
- IV. Bags
- V. Accessories
- VI. Customized vehicles and vans with a lift
- VII. Miscellaneous equipment
- VIII. Additional equipment and information
    - a. ____
    - b. ____

The individual and the primary caregiver should take time before an item is purchased to understand the purpose and the need for the equipment. It is important to understand the following:

1. Purpose for the equipment.
    a. Always consider the individual needs, activities, and the options in style and color.
2. Do you need a prescription?
3. Cost and optional items available.
4. Check with insurance or any other service regarding as follows:
    a. Coverage of the purchase and the type of co-pay.
    b. Frequency of replacement (generally, every two years or after a surgery).
5. Who handles any repairs?
6. What are the safety considerations?
7. Ask your physician for a mobility service provider referral.
    a. Equipment orders and repairs are generally through a mobility service provider. When personalizing this section, be sure to state the maintenance and where it can be serviced, cleaned, and any pertinent information.

I. WHEELCHAIR

1. A prescription from your physician is required for coverage by your insurance.
2. Request reevaluation assessments every two to three years to ensure that the equipment continues to adequately meet the appropriate needs.
3. Work with the mobility specialist to ensure the proper fit, chair height, and balance.
4. Manual, sports, and power chairs—There are various designs to meet your independent style of activity and use. It will be important to inform the mobility specialist on your type of activities to ensure the accuracy of the evaluation.
5. When ordering, discuss these important areas with the specialist:
    a. Solid frame versus folding chair (ask about the pros and cons).
    b. Balance and comfort.
    c. Shoulder placement and the center point to the wheel axle. Ensure that the hands maneuver the wheels easily on a manual chair. Correct placement may require various adjustments.
    d. The sitting height, including the cushion of the chair, needs consideration to ensure that a person can fit comfortably under most tables.
    e. Seat belt is an important safety feature and required if using public transportation or a transport service while sitting in the chair.
    f. Back of chair height.
        i. Sports chairs generally have a lower back height. It is important to ensure safety and security while maintaining balance and comfort.
6. Power chairs require checking the battery daily for charging and maintenance. Use the manufacturer's guidelines for the proper care.
    a. Be sure to ask how to transport. Can it be taken apart easily, and what form of vehicle transportation is recommended?
    b. Will it require a van and a lift purchase? If so, see number VII. Miscellaneous Equipment for guidelines.
7. Seat
    a. The knee edge of the seat length should have a two-finger space from behind the knee to minimize the chance of reduced leg and feet circulation, as well as proper leg and foot placement.
    b. The seat width needs appropriate space for comfort and stability.
        i. Consider the distance of the arm reach with manual chairs to have proper shoulder extension while wheeling.
    c. The correct angle can provide stability, balance, and comfort. This is important when a chair is ordered.

i. Too much of a seating angle (a.k.a. bucket angle) can cause problems by adding pressure to the blood supply and nerves that can affect balance.
   - A bucket refers to the seat angle between the front and back that can vary by specific degrees.

ii. Discuss the options and how it will best meet your needs.

iii. Sports or daily activity may have an effect on the degree angle.

8. Small front-wheel casters: The size and type of wheel can make a difference in maneuverability.
9. Tires
   a. There are several <u>types</u> of tires, wheel sizes, and camber angles to consider for maneuverability. Some of the areas to consider are as follows:
      i. Shoulder extension
      ii. Balance
      iii. Height for your leg and feet position and table height
      iv. Many individuals find that having a camber angled allows for easy maneuverability especially for sports activities.
         - Be sure to watch the camber angled in order to fit in doorways.
      v. Always ask your mobility specialist for more considerations.
         ➢ **<u>Note:</u>**
            - Using tube liners will help prevent flat tires or ask your dealer for other alternatives.
            - Tires should be checked frequently by the caregiver to maintain good air pressure.
            - Side of tire will tell you the appropriate air pressure.
            - You can purchase tires through the wheelchair provider or at a bike shop.
10. Accessories (Optional)
   a. Ask what is available.
   b. Arm rest
      i Some people feel it interferes with pushing and the style or sleekness they want.
      ii. Push handles can be attached or are part of the back of the frame.
   c. Antitip wheels are attached to the bottom of the back of the chair to help prevent tipping and may be required on some transport vehicles.
11. Specialized equipment attached to a chair requires individual training and manufacturer's guidelines. Add what care is required to your *Personal Care Handbook* and the *Personal Caregiver Handbook*.

12. It can be exciting once you find out that the item you have waited for finally arrives so it is easy to overlook what may be very important. Therefore, be sure to check and review the following:
    a. All the areas that are important for you and the order to ensure that you received the product you wanted the way you want it.
    b. Proper balance and comfort.
    c. Ensure that the wheelchair will not tip backward easily. If it does, it may require the following:
        i Antitip wheels to prevent falling. Check with the mobility specialist to ensure you are safe and comfortable.
        ii. The wheel axle plate placement to adjust the chair balance.
        iii. The height of the caster wheels may need adjusting.

II. CUSHIONS: General Information

1. It is very important to request an experienced seating specialist to assist you with proper seating evaluation assessments. You will need a prescription from your physician.
2. Generally, cushions are made of various materials. They can include a combination of products, such as foam, gel packs, honeycomb, and air cells. If you have an allergy to latex or another foam product, it will be very important to notify the service provider.
3. The purpose of a properly fitted back and seating cushion provides the following:
    a. Balance and comfort
    b. Better positioning and seating posture
    c. To help prevent decubitus sores
    d. To provide comfort as using the seating sling of the wheelchair can become uncomfortable when sitting for any length of time, making a properly fitted cushion necessary
4. It is important to check for any hard surfaces that may be touching any part of the back or buttock areas as it could create a sore. Discuss with your seating specialist or physician.
5. Cushion and wheelchair reevaluation
    a. Check with your insurance provider regarding the replacement frequency for your equipment.
    b. Generally, the reassessment can be a minimum of every two to three years or after a surgery that can affect your needs.

A. Seating cushion

1. The purpose is for comfort, balance, leg and feet placement, and to help prevent decubitus sores.

2. Consult a seating specialist to evaluate if a special seating cushion is required to accommodate the needs caused by pressure areas or medical concerns.
3. Things to be considered in the evaluation:
    a. Request a pressure evaluation to ensure that the cushion recommended provides the best support. It may be necessary to evaluate various types of cushions.
    b. Shoulder placement—are they balanced while using the chair? Is the individual balanced in all aspects of the chair and its use?
    c. Be sure there is a two-finger space between the back of the knee and the edge of the cushion. This helps body-seating placement, to prevent blood clots, and leg pressure.
    d. Cushion height can increase the overall chair height. Consider table height comfort when at a normal height table for meals, work, and school; in the car, you need to consider the roof if the head is touching, etc.
4. Be sure cushion cover is clean and fits correctly—*no* gaps or bulges.
    a. The manufacturer can supply additional zippered covers for an additional cost.
    b. I have purchased material and had a cover made with elastic so it is easy to change and wash. Not only is this economical, but it is also nice when the material is personalized.
    c. The removable seat cover should be changed at least once a day or when soiled. (Note: it may appear clean, but you could notice a strong odor.)
    d. White vinegar acts as an antibacterial to help remove odor and to clean with laundry.
5. In cleaning a soiled cushion, consider the following:
    a. CHECK THE MANUFACTURER'S BOOKLET FOR THEIR CLEANING RECOMMENDATIONS.
    b. **<u>DO NOT WASH UNLESS IT IS STATED ON THE CUSHION.</u>**
    c. The majority of cushions have a removable zippered cover. Clean as directed.
    d. If there are no instructions available and no removable cover, you can gentle clean with soft cloth.
        i. Use mild soap, adding a little white vinegar to your water. White vinegar acts as an antibacterial to help remove odor and clean.
        ii. Baking soda also can help with cleaning and odor. Note: Do not use the baking soda and the vinegar together as it can undesirably produce foam that is similar to a science experiment. There are cleaning products specially designed to minimize or eliminate odor available through medical suppliers.
            - You can check with your insurance for coverage when you place an order for incontinent products.

- These products are generally designed for any plastic, such as tubing or any type of leg bags as it minimizes breaking down of the product.

iii. Remove most of the moisture with a damp cloth.

iv. Pat dry with towel, and use a hair dryer if needed.

6. Cushion or wheelchair odor
   a. This can be embarrassing for the person using the chair. It would be best to find the source and clean as soon as possible.
   b. In the event you experience a problem when you are away from your home, you can maintain the dignity of the individual from embarrassment by being prepared. Keeping something in the vehicle like the following can help:
      - Additional covers and clothing
      - Lysol spray to disinfect
      - Nonscented air freshener or cologne
      - Or something you may find that works better

B. Back cushion. Generally, this is special ordered through a seating specialist.

1. The purpose of this is for back protection, lower back support, balance, and seating comfort.
2. Be sure that it fits properly and attached appropriately.

III. SHOWER CHAIR

1. Recommend a long padded chair that allows for stability and better balance.
2. If staying at a hotel, call ahead and ask what type of shower chair they have available to assure that it will work to meet your individual needs for balance, stability, and safety.
3. Take a portable travel shower chair to ensure stability when away from home. There are portable shower chairs available online that are lightweight and easy to transport. Taking your own chair helps to ensure stability, safety, comfort, and independence.
4. You may need to use both the hotel's shower chair and your portable shower chair depending on the accessibility needed for transferring or for an additional seating area.

IV. BAGS. See Personal Bags Organization section for more information.

1. A backpack should generally carry personal supplies and spare clothes.
2. A side pack or an under-chair pack holds personal belongings:
   a. Wallet
   b. Keys
   c. Etc.
3. Phone pack.

a. Attach to the side of chair.
b. Phone bag should be waterproof type.
c. Has a closure to minimize any water exposure.
d. Phone is always charged and ready for usage. (This is for a caregiver to check.)

V. ACCESSORIES. Look on the Internet for wheelchairs, cushions, and accessories.

1. Emergency alert button (optional)
    a. Check the equipment as stated on the instruction sheet.
    b. Check periodically to be sure it works and if it requires new batteries or charging.

VI. CUSTOMIZED VEHICLES AND VANS WITH A LIFT

1. There are several service dealers available. You will need to check in your area.
2. Be careful with the door height to ensure that the person sitting in the chair can fit through the height opening; an expanded top may be required.
3. Vehicles can be equipped with hand controls. A therapist can assist with more information.
4. It will be important to work with a driver training instruction specialist for disabled individuals to understand how to drive with the adaptive equipment safely.
5. It would be best to understand how to repair some of the equipment and what to do if a problem occurs (i.e., the lift will not move, etc.).
6. When purchasing a new vehicle many times, a dealership may provide a credit for adaptive equipment. Check with your dealership on the dollar allowance and if they will do the modification.

VII. MISCELLANEOUS EQUIPMENT

1. It would be best to speak with your physician, occupational and physical therapist, the mobility provider regarding equipment to best assist you and what is recommended for your mobility and safety, such as follows:
    a. Walkers—there are many styles. Check with your mobility provider or therapist as one style may appear more portable or offer additional benefits, but it may not be the right one. It may be a safety hazard that you are not aware of and can affect your balance.
    b. There are many types of products available, and it would be helpful to research the product for your specific needs. Your local medical supplier will have booklets and products for you to consider.

VIII. Additional Equipment and Information

NOTE: Add additional information needed for your individual needs and living style.

Equipment Maintenance Fill In

CONTACT 1. Primary caregiver ❑ See list ________________ Phone ________________________

2. Mobility service provider ____________________ Contact ______________________

Phone ____________________________ E-mail __________________________________

Address ____

____

The individual and the primary caregiver should take time before an item is purchased to understand the purpose and the need for the equipment. *Make a copy of this form for each item.*

Item____Date______________

1. Purpose
   a. ____
   b. ____
   c. ____
2. Do you need a prescription? ❑ YES ❑ NO
   a. Doctor____ Phone_______________
   b. ____
3. Funding ❑ Insurance ❑ Regional Center ❑ Self ❑ Other
   a. Purchase coverage ____
   b. Co-pay ____
   c. Frequency of replacement ____
4. Who handles any repairs?
   a. ____
5. What are the safety considerations? ❑ See attached
   a. ____
   b. ____
6. Maintenance and care ❑ See attached
   a. ____
   b. ____
   c. ____
7. Accessories (optional)
   a. ____
   b. ____

8. Description ❑ See attached

 Color________ Fabric________ Height______ Length______ Width______ Weight______

 a. ____

 b. ____

9. Transportation (If applicable)

 ❑ Fits in current vehicle ❑ Modifications to vehicle required ❑ New vehicle required

 ❑ Meets public transportation standards

 a. ____

 b. ____

10. ❑ Reevaluation assessments ❑ Repair ❑ Other ______________________________

 a. Date____

  Comment____

  ____

 b. Date____

  Comment____

  ____

 c. Date____

  Comment____

  ____

<u>CUSHION OR SEATING</u>

A. Seating cushion

 a. Date____

  ❑ Replace ❑ Repair ❑ Cleaning frequency______________________________

  ____

 b. Date____

  ❑ Replace ❑ Repair ❑ Cleaning frequency______________________________

  ____

B. Special Instructions ❑ See attached

 a. CHECK THE MANUFACTURER'S BOOKLET FOR THEIR CLEANING RECOMMENDATIONS.

 b. ❑ Wash removable cover____

 c. ❑ Cleaning instructions____

 d. ❑____

<u>NOTE</u>: Add additional information needed for your individual needs and living style.

8
Home Care Facilities and Independent Living

In the context of this handbook a home care facility can also represent a group home depending on your location and what they may call a home that is run by an agency or privately to care for a disabled individual.

Budget and Independent Living Needs

This can assist you with your budgeting needs. Be sure to add any additional financial information.

Home Care Questionnaire

This gives you a basic list of questions to consider when searching for a care facility. There are many options available so it is important to check the various homes to see what they offer in services, safety considerations, cleanliness, and type of inner action between the consumers and the attendants. You can search various Web sites that offer additional information.

Independent Living Property Search

This provides some areas to consider when looking for property. You may want to take picture on your cell phone or camera for reference. Be sure to add your own questions. Review and check the local services to ensure that your needs are conveniently accessible.

Resources to Search

There are various organizations and Web sites to research, and consider all options for any age as the information offered can assist by offering valuable resourceful information when you need to consider living outside of the home. Some programs offer a complete support team that you will need to ask what is involved and always what the cost could be. They sometimes will take what funding sources you may have and social security checks to cover all or most of the living expenses so it is very important to ask what is offered and the expense that may be incurred.

Also if you are considering home care, ask what occurs if the individual has an anger or violent temper situation, gets sick, or has a wound of some kind that requires dressing changes. This is important as some of these homes will not take a person if nursing care is needed. So be sure to ask that if a situation occurs, what are the steps that you will need to know should they release the individual quickly. Hopefully, you will not have to deal with this, but it can occur and it is best to be aware in the event something happens.

Some of the resources or subject search areas to consider are to speak with your social worker from your funding programs, hospital, and various organizations you participate in; the Web offers a wide range of options and is a good place to research—examples are AARP, group or home care, the local Regional Center may have a home care, etc. if you qualify. Some of the online Web sites may require to search deeper within the site to find what you are looking for or to call their contact number listed.

Budget and Independent Living Needs

DATE_________________

This can assist you with your budgeting needs. Be sure to add any additional financial information.

1. ❑ Apartment ❑ Home

Address_________________________________City__________ST__________Zip__________

Rent Total $___ Mo. ❑ Lease: ❑ Month to Month ❑ 3 Mos. ❑ 6 Mos. ❑ 9 Mos. ❑ 12 Mos.

❑ Other____

Deposit $____________

a. ❑ Pay: ❑ Electricity ❑ Phone ❑ Cable TV ❑ Garbage ❑ Water ❑ Other

b. ❑ Downstairs ❑ Upstairs ❑ Elevators ❑ Meets ADA Requirements

c. ❑ Larger Kitchen ❑ Lower Countertops ❑ Wider Doorways

d. ❑ Bedroom Fits Furniture ❑ Bathroom Wheelchair Accessible (if needed)

e. ❑ Laundry: Washer/Dryer ❑ Inside ❑ On Property ❑ Not Available ❑Laundromat

2. ROOMMATE ❑ Individual ❑ Renter/Tenant Rents Room ❑ Caregiver

a. Rent ❑ $_______Monthly ❑ $________Bimonthly

b. ❑ Discount Rent Explain_____________________________________

c. Paid by ❑ Renter ❑ Personal Funds ❑ Family ❑ Other:

❑ Service Agency____

d. ❑ Be financially responsible to the apartment management.

❑ Credit Check____

e. Bills responsible for ❑ ½ Utilities ❑ Electricity ❑ TV ❑ Water ❑ Garbage ❑ % Phone

❑ Other____

3. CASE MANAGER ❑ Hourly $_________ ❑ Weekly $_________ ❑ Monthly $______________

a. Paid by ❑ Personal Funds ❑ Family ❑ Service Agency

4. CAREGIVER ❑ Hourly $_________ ❑ Weekly $_________ ❑ Monthly $________________

a. Paid by ❑ Personal Funds ❑ Family ❑ Service Agency______________________________

b. Funding Sources for Caregiver

❑____ ❑ Hours Monthly__________

❑____ ❑ Hours Monthly__________

5. INDIVIDUAL'S BUDGET SUMMARY

a. Monthly Income

Wages $ _________

SSI $ _________

SSD $ ________
Disability $ ________
Roommate $ ________
________________ $ ________
________________ $ ________
________________ $ ________
Total Income **$** ________

b. Monthly Expenses

Rent $ ________ ❑ Full ❑ __ % of bill ❑ Other
TV/Internet $ ________ ❑ Full ❑ __ % of bill ❑ Other
Phone $ ________ ❑ Cell ❑ Personal ❑ Other
Electricity $ ________ ❑ Full ❑ __ % of bill ❑ Other
Groceries $ ________
Transportation $ ________ ❑ Outreach ❑ Taxi ❑ Bus Pass
Recreation/Leisure $ ________ ❑ Movies ❑ Outings ❑ Other
________________ $ ________ *Explain* ________________________
________________ $ ________ *Explain* ________________________
Total Expenses **$** ________

c. Medical expenses

<u>Medical Coverage</u> $ ________ ❑ Monthly Insurance
Share of Cost $ ________
Co-pay $ ________
Out of Pocket expense $ ________
Total Estimated Medical **$** ________
❑ Medical ❑ Dental ❑ Vision & Hearing ❑ Other ________________________
Funding Sources: ❑ Private Insurance ❑ Medi-Cal/Other ❑ Medicare ❑ Personal Funds
❑ Other ____

<u>Prescriptions</u> $ ________ ❑ Monthly Insurance
Share of Cost $ ________
Co-pay $ ________
Out of pocket expense $ ________
Total Estimated Prescriptions $________
Funding Sources: ❑ Private Insurance ❑ Medi-Cal/Other ❑ Medicare ❑ Personal Funds
❑ Other ____

d. Total Income Expenses

Total Income	$ ________	
Total Expenses	$ -________	
Total Medical Expenses	$ -________	
Caregiver	$ -________	Paid by ❑ Individual ❑ Family ❑ Agency
Case Manager	$ -________	Paid by ❑ Individual ❑ Family ❑ Agency
Other	$ -________	
Total	**$** ________	
Any Outstanding Total	**$** ________	*Who will cover this portion?*

6. Additional Information

Home Care Questionnaire

DATE____________________

This gives you a basic list of questions to consider when searching for a care facility. There are many options available so it is important to check the various homes to see what they offer in services, safety considerations, cleanliness, and type of inner action between the consumers and the attendants. You can search various Web sites that offer additional information. Take pictures of the outside, inside, the bedrooms, and bathrooms for your reference, you can use your cell phone

Business name____

Address ____________________________________City__________________ St____ Zip____

Phone__________________________________ Fax_________________ Cell_______________

Web Site____________________________________ E-mail______________________________

Contact____ Title/Position_______________

Business License No.____________________________Certificate License No.________________

Type Business Licenses____

Number of years in business: Facility_________Person offering service___________________

Number of employees assisting___________ P/T_____F/T_____Are they licensed? ❑ YES ❑ NO

Number of consumers___________ No. of males___________ No. of females___________

Type of disabilities____

Age range of consumers______________Other expectations____________________________

____

FACILITY

Number of bedrooms: ❑ single rooms_________ ❑ shared rooms__________

Number of consumers per room: ❑ 2 ❑ 3 ❑ _________ Size of bedrooms______________

Number of bathrooms:________ ❑ private____ ❑ shared____ ❑ How many consumers per bathroom?________

FEE SCHEDULE Per month $______________ Accepts: ❑ SSI______ ❑ IHSS______

❑ Other____

HOME CARE RESPONSIBILITIES. Use the back or separate page for additional concerns and your notes.

❑ Case manager

- ❑ Personal care attendants
- ❑ Laundry
- ❑ Cleaning room
- ❑ Distribute medication
- ❑ Orders prescriptions
- ❑ Reorders prescriptions
- ❑ Orders Nondurable Items (i.e., pads, ostomy, catheters, diapers/briefs, etc.)
- ❑ Meal preparation/special diets
- ❑ Groceries: Who purchases favorite items and how are they purchased?
- ❑ Furniture in room Use their own, i.e.,
- ❑ Bed
- ❑ TV
- ❑ Dresser
- ❑ Other
- ❑ Cell phone
- ❑ Phone in room/own (self-pay)
- ❑ Privacy__________________
- ❑ Other____________

EXIT/LEAVE REQUIREMENTS

Type ❑ Overnight/Weekend visit ❑ Extended visit ❑ Leave facility permanently

Notice_________ How many days/hours prior?________ Penalty fees? Explain.________________

Away from facility: ❑ Day Trips ❑ Vacations ❑ Illness ❑ Limitations:______________________

If a medical situation occurs, what is your policy?______________________________________

1. Must leave the facility immediately? ❑ NO ❑ YES (*Explain*)______________________
2. Allowed to return while recovering? ❑ NO ❑ YES (*Explain*)______________________
3. Allowed to return after recovery? ❑ NO ❑ YES (*Explain*)______________________

Additional information____

Independent Living Property Search

DATE___________________

This provides some areas to consider when looking for property. You may want to take pictures on your cell phone or camera for reference. Be sure to add your own questions. Review and check the local services to ensure that your needs are conveniently accessible.

Location

Address____ City_________ ST____ Zip____
Contact____ Phone______________________
Web site____ E-mail_____________________
When available_______________________________________

❑ Ground floor ❑ Other floors ❑ No.________ ❑ No. of elevators_______ Notes_____________

Rent ❑ Monthly $________ ❑ Deposit $_______ ❑ Additional costs $________ Explain_______

Lease ❑ Monthly ❑ 6 Months ❑ 12 Months ❑ Other ______________________________

No. of Bedrooms________ Baths accessible? ❑ NO ❑ YES ❑ Shower door and space width accessible? ❑ Tub

Laundry ❑ NO ❑ YES ❑ W/D hookup Inside ❑ Electric or ❑ Gas ❑ Facility: Cost of machines per wash/dry_______

Furnished: ❑ NO ❑ YES ❑ Full ❑ Partial ❑ Other_____________________________

Willing to allow adaptions? ❑ NO ❑ YES Type_______________________________

Any limitations or conditions? ❑ NO ❑ YES_______________________________

❑ Low cupboards (especially important for wheelchair accessibility)

Utilities included	❑ Electric	❑ NO ❑ YES	❑ Gas	❑ NO ❑ YES
	Water	❑ NO ❑ YES		
	Garbage	❑ NO ❑ YES		
	Cable	❑ NO ❑ YES (Check where the outlet/s is located)		
	Phone Line	❑ NO ❑ YES (Check where the outlet/s is located)		
	Other ______________________________			

Parking: ❑ NO ❑ YES. If yes, where do you park vehicles? ❑ Handicap Space ❑ Garage ❑ Stall ❑ Costs______

Check the areas that the property offers

❑ Swimming pool ❑ Spa ❑ Exercise room ❑ Clubhouse/social area ❑ Other_______________

❑ Ramps ❑ Railing ❑ Accessible to other areas of property ❑ Other____________________

Property/neighborhood appear ❑ Safe ❑ Clean ❑ Nice ❑ Other_______________________

Security ❑ Gated ❑ Patrol on Duty: ❑ NO ❑ YES ❑ Daily ❑ Evenings ❑ Other___________

Do the hallways and stairways provide easy access when moving furniture? ❑ NO ❑ YES

Additional Information____

Near

Bus Stop: ❑ YES Bus No._____❑ NO Distance to nearest bus stop________________________

Shopping: ❑ YES ❑ NO Distance to nearest stores_______ Type ❑ Grocery ❑ Other_________

Bank: ❑ YES Type____________ ❑ NO Distance to nearest bank_________________________

Entertainment: ❑ NO ❑ YES Type____

Notes ____ ❑ See additional notes

9
Medical Concerns Checklist

When an illness or medical condition occurs, this section describes how the caregiver can best assist the individual; it is also helpful for the medical team when an emergency arises. It will be important that all information is thoroughly documented and kept up to date. There is a separate fill-in section of this form for you to customize to meet your needs.

As the origin of the needs attached to the sample form pertain mostly to an individual with spina bifida, it may have areas that do not pertain to your specific needs. Simply change any or all areas in order to meet your individual needs.

Take this with you when an emergency situation occurs or if there is a medical situation that you have been having a problem to find a solution. This form has been well received and helpful to the medical team, especially in an emergency situation when they are working to eliminate a particular diagnosis to find the appropriate treatment. It has eliminated specific testing and expedited in locating a treatment.

It also gives the medical team the confidence of the "team approach," and they generally welcome your ideas and assistance easier.

Medical Concerns Checklist

Name____Date______________

CONTACT 1. Primary caregiver ❑ See list______________________________ Phone______________

2. Physician ❑ See list____________________________________ Phone______________

➢ Notify the primary caregiver or the physician immediately if you notice an illness, condition, or an abnormality.

WHEN AN ILLNESS OR CONDITION OCCURS, HERE ARE AREAS TO CONSIDER.

There are separate sections regarding each area with more explicit information to assist you.

A. REMEMBER—If you need to go to the doctor or the emergency room, take the following:

a. *Personal Medical Journal* or *Medical History Summary*
b. Medical supply bag with the individual's specific incontinence and/or personal items, especially nonlatex items if there is a latex allergy.
c. *Personal Care Handbook* that includes specific personal information or the Medical Concerns Checklist.
d. Any X-rays to assist a medical professional that is located_____________________________.

IMPORTANT: DO NOT LEAVE ANY X-RAYS OR REPORTS AT THE HOSPITAL OR AT PHYSICIANS OFFICE!

B. VOMITING. Always be alert for other symptoms that may be part of this situation.

a. ____
b. ____

C. BLOOD PRESSURE and HEART RATE

a. Normal is approximately 120/80. Individual's normal is______________________
b. If elevated, check all areas in this Medical Concerns Checklist section for possible reasons for the elevation.

D. FEVER. Notify the primary caregiver and/or the physician immediately

a. Individual's normal temperature is approximately___________________________
b. Anything above normal warrants to check for a medical condition such as a (UTI) urinary tract infection, decubitus, broken bones, infections, etc.
c. ____

E. CONCERN AREAS. The following areas have corresponding numbers to the pages when the form is printed that provides additional pertinent information:

1. **ALLERGIES ❑ Medication ❑ Food ❑**__________ See Page________
2. **DECUBITUS** See Page________

3. **SEIZURES** See Page_______
4. **STROKE IDENTIFICATION** See Page_______
5. **URINARY TRACT INFECTION** See Page_______
6. **VOMITING** See Page_______
7. **SHUNTS** See Page_______
8. **ARNOLD CHIARI** See Page_______
9. ________________________________ See Page_______

1. ALLERGIES

CONTACT 1. Primary caregiver ❑ See list ______________________________ Phone __________

2. Physician ❑ See list ____________________________________ Phone __________

➢ Notify the primary caregiver or the physician immediately if you notice an illness, condition, or an abnormality.

• **SEE MEDICATION AND FOOD ALLERGY LIST.** If additional information is needed, add another sheet.

i. **Medication** ❑ See additional list

A. TYPE____

1. Symptom____
2. Remedy____
   a. Medication____
   b. How to assist____
   c. ____

B. TYPE____

1. Symptom____
2. Remedy____
   a. Medication____
   b. How to assist____
   c. ____

ii. **Foods** ❑ See additional list

A. TYPE____

1. Symptom____
2. Remedy____
   a. Medication____
   b. How to assist____
   c. ____

B. TYPE____

1. Symptom____
2. Remedy____
   a. Medication____
   b. How to assist____
   c. ____

2. DECUBITUS, BEDSORES, BURNS

CONTACT 1. Primary caregiver ❑ See list ______________________ Phone __________

2. Physician ❑ See list ______________________ Phone __________

➢ Notify the primary caregiver or the physician immediately if you notice an illness, condition, or an abnormality.

• The physician will need to see the patient and may refer care to a wound care specialist.

A. Symptoms

a. Vomiting
b. Fever
c. Open wound
d. Skin discoloration at wound site
e. Other (Explain)______________________

B. Check body

a. Feet, especially for burn blisters, i.e., water too hot in shower, infections, or poor circulation.
b. Legs, especially for burn blisters, i.e., water too hot in shower, placing hot items on thighs, prolonged computer laptop use if resting on legs, exposure to sun, any type of open wound, or infection.
c. Buttock area for discoloration, any type of open wound or infection.
d. Arm and elbow area for possible sores or burn blisters.
e. Fingers for possible blisters, any injuries or sores from pushing a wheelchair, walker, etc.
f. Private area for an infection, yeast infection, or decubitus ulcers.
g. Bruises, open wounds.
h. Other (Explain)______________________

C. Wounds

a. Be sure to follow the instructions of your physician or the wound care specialist.
b. When you first identify a wound, be sure to cover with some type of light bandage.
c. Do not put any pressure on the wound area.
d. Monitor the wound area when sitting or lying and observe how the body comes in contact with any pressure area.
e. Check with your insurance carrier; you may have medical coverage for wound care supplies. You will have to obtain a prescription from your physician in most cases. Be sure to ask where to obtain supplies.
f. Assess what wound supplies you may have at home in case a new or reorder is necessary.
g. When calling the medical supplier, be sure to mention you are handling a wound and need the order quickly.

D. Cleaning of wound area

a. Follow the direction of your physician or wound care specialist.

E. General information

a. Remember there should be no hard contact with the injured area.
b. Use a light sheet to cover if the wound is on the buttocks or private area to maintain the dignity of the individual.
c. Ask the specialist for all other instructions, such as if they are able to take a shower, travel, sit, etc.

F. Progression of wound healing generally observed. Check with the specialist for more information.

1. White layer
2. Pink layer
3. Bloody (good, means circulation is establishing)
4. Edges become smaller
5. Repeat of numbers 1–4 above until healed
6. Continually prompt and monitor to stay off the area.
7. Ask your physician if the following would be recommended:
    - An increase level of zinc has been known to improve skin redevelopment. (Be sure to discuss with physician prior to increasing zinc so there is no conflict with treatment or medication. Zinc can be taken orally or used topically.)
    - Protein food or nutrients has been recognized as a good source for tissue redevelopment.

G. Travel. When going to the doctor or hospital, see Community Transportation, Section 6.

a. If you have latex allergies, take all nonlatex products in your medical travel bag with personal items, any applicable X-rays, and notebook or binder with caregiver notes, especially the Daily Vitals Record Keeping that includes the blood pressure and temperature.

H. Follow-up

a. Everyone who is working with the client will need to have the instructions for proper care from the doctor or wound care specialist and from your notes.
b. Visiting nursing staff may be required to come in periodically to check the wound, dressing, and make any recommendations.

I. Prevention techniques

a. Cushions for wheelchairs and other seating devices:
   1. Fitting is appropriate.
   2. Placement is appropriate.
      a. Back
         - Should be secured to back of chair and not worn down.
         - See Equipment Maintenance section for proper seating, fitting, and maintenance.
      b. Seat
         - Should not show excessive wear.
         - Should not have a hard or uneven surface that could create a decubitus sore.
   3. Fabric
      a. Securely on cushions
      b. Changed and washed daily or when soiled
   4. Transfers. Watch how individual transfers in and out of chair.
      a. Is the body hitting or rubbing anything that could create a sore?
      b. Be sure to advise the client as they may not realize they are creating a sore or understand the importance of an alternative transfer method.
   5. Bedding. Monitor the bedding to ensure it is free of wrinkles and bulk, secured well, and the bottom area of the bedding is flat.

3. SEIZURES

CONTACT 1. Primary caregiver ❑ See list ______________________________ Phone __________

2. Physician ❑ See list ____________________________________ Phone __________

➢ Notify the primary caregiver or the physician immediately if you notice an illness, condition, or an abnormality.

✶ **NOTE:** *Do not give* any Tylenol, aspirin, or ibuprofen-type medication. This can mask a symptom if there is a serious medical condition.

A. **Symptoms**. These are some symptoms to be able to distinguish a seizure. You may have other information as symptoms are different for each individual.

a. Discoloration of skin: purplish or whitish.

b. Disoriented:

   1. Speech sluggish or verbiage is not clear
   2. Unable to stay with a conversation.
   3. Appears on some type of drug.

c. Eyes fixed or strange movements.

d. Shaking of the body.

e. If the person has a shunt, it could represent an additional problem.

B. **Concerns**

a. Check each area of the Medical Concerns Checklist section for possibilities of medical problems that could cause the seizure.

b. It could be the possibility of medication reaction that affects blood levels.

c. When taking to doctor or hospital, see Community Transportation Section 7.

d. If you have latex allergies, take all nonlatex products, medical travel bag with personal items, any applicable X-rays, and notebook or binder with caregiver notes, especially the Daily Care Log that includes the blood pressure and temperature.

C. **Follow-up**

Everyone working with the individual will need to have the instructions on how to handle future seizures.

D. **Additional information**

____

____

____

____

____

____

4. STROKE IDENTIFICATION

If he or she has trouble with ANY ONE of the following tasks, call emergency immediately and describe**.**

Sometimes symptoms of a stroke are difficult to identify. Unfortunately, the lack of awareness spells disaster. The stroke victim may suffer severe brain damage when people fail to recognize the symptoms of a stroke.

Now, doctors say YOU can recognize a stroke by asking three simple questions:

S - Ask the individual to SMILE.
T - Ask the person to TALK and SPEAK A SIMPLE SENTENCE (coherently) for example, "It is sunny out today" and person is unable to stay focused in the conversation.
R - Ask them to RAISE BOTH ARMS.

Another sign of a stroke: "Stick **O**ut Your Tongue"

- Ask the person to stick out his tongue.
- If the tongue is crooked or if it goes to one side or the other, that is also an indication of a stroke.

You may want to include additional information.

This is a situation that could have been prevented.

During a BBQ, a woman stumbled and took a little fall; she assured everyone that she was fine (they offered to call paramedics). She said she had just tripped over a brick because of her new shoes.

They got her cleaned up and got her a new plate of food. While she appeared a bit shaken up, Jane went about enjoying herself the rest of the evening.

Jane's husband called later, telling everyone that his wife had been taken to the hospital. At 6:00 p.m., Jane passed away. She had suffered a stroke at the BBQ.

Had they known how to identify the signs of a stroke, perhaps Jane would be with us today. Some don't die. They can end up in a helpless, hopeless condition instead.

A neurologist says that if he can get to a stroke victim within three hours, he can hopefully reverse the effects of a stroke totally. He said the trick was getting a stroke recognized, diagnosed, and then getting the patient medically cared for within three hours, which can be the difficult part.

This information is to assist you and a collection from several sources.

5. URINARY TRACT INFECTION (UTI)

CONTACT 1. Primary caregiver ❑ See list ______________________________ Phone ___________

2. Physician ❑ See list ____________________________________ Phone ___________

➢ Notify the primary caregiver or the physician immediately if you notice an illness, condition, or an abnormality.

A. **SYMPTOMS**

a. Blood in urine (pain, spasms, or discomfort).
b. Smell, strong odor (can indicate an infection).
   1. Noticeable as soon as you enter the room or surroundings.
   2. Stools will also have a stronger odor.
c. Vomiting.
d. Fever.
e. Irritability.
f. Blood pressure increase or decrease.
g. Lethargy.
h. Back pain on either the left or right side may generally indicate a kidney infection.

B. **URINE ANALYSIS (UA)**

a. Bloody.
b. It is important to take a urine sample to the doctor's office or a designated laboratory to establish the type of bacteria for the proper diagnosis, medication, and to ensure the appropriate treatment.
c. Write instructions on how to obtain a urine sample, which would be best handled for the individual or the physician will be able to give you explicit instructions to follow.
   - The (UA) urine specimen container should be placed in a baggie to prevent leakage with the individual's name and date.
   - The UA should be placed in a brown lunch bag with the name on the outside.
   - Then it should be placed in the refrigerator, or placed on ice, to prevent bacteria growth until it is taken immediately from the refrigerator to the physician or laboratory.

C. **MAKE AN APPOINTMENT AS SOON AS POSSIBLE**.

a. Be sure to pack any incontinence products to include latex-free products if applicable:
   - Diapers (briefs), pads, and/or catheters
   - Gloves
   - Wallet with insurance card, credit card, checkbook, or cash to pay the doctor
   - Assist as needed

Note: An outreach transportation service can require twenty-four (24) hour notice.

D. **FOLLOW-UP**. Find out if there is a bacterial infection and what treatment is recommended.

a. The doctor will give instructions as to what is needed, be sure to ask when the results will be available.

b. It will be important to follow up with a phone call or to check online for the results. Do not depend on a callback from the doctor's office.

c. If a prescription is necessary,

   1. check against the allergy listing,
   2. give the doctor's office your pharmacy number or location,
   3. pick up the medication.

d. When you pick up the medication, check to ensure it is what has been prescribed by the physician.

   1. It is recommended to keep all medication in a medication tray to ensure that it is distributed appropriately.
   2. Notify the primary caregiver immediately upon onset of any complications or if you notice that the medication appears to be correcting the symptoms in a timely manner.

E. **RECHECK**. Be sure to ask the doctor if they need any of the following:

a. To have another urinalysis to ensure that the infection has been eliminated.

b. Another appointment. If so,

   1. schedule the appointment and
   2. contact outreach for transportation if applicable.

F. **ADDITIONAL INFORMATION**

6. VOMITING

❑ This can be an indication of other concerns that need to be checked, such as the flu or another diagnosis.

CONTACT 1. Primary caregiver ❑ See list ______________________ Phone __________

2. Physician ❑ See list ___________________________ Phone __________

➢ Notify the primary caregiver or the physician immediately if you notice an illness, condition, or an abnormality.

A. SYMPTOMS

a. Vomiting

1. Frequency____

2. Color ❑ Food ❑ Blood ❑ Phlegm

3. ❑ Note____

____

____

B. HOW TO HANDLE

❑ Call doctor____

❑ Emergency ❑ Immediately ❑ Monitor____________________

❑ Medication Type______________ Dosage__________ Frequency__________

❑ Other

____

____

____

____

____

____

____

____

____

____

____

7. SHUNTS

❑ See additional sections with more information.

CONTACT 1. Primary caregiver ❑ See list ______________________________ Phone ___________

2. Physician ❑ See list ____________________________________ Phone ___________

➢ Notify the primary caregiver or the physician immediately if you notice an illness, condition, or an abnormality.

A. **SYMPTOMS.** It will be best to list the symptoms you want to ensure are monitored by your physician.

❑ Headache ❑ Eye sensitivity to light ❑ Cognitive speech is unclear

❑ Red tracking on neck and chest areas ❑ Swelling around tubing area

❑ The ophthalmologist can check to see if there is pressure on the optic nerve.

❑ ____

❑ ____

❑ ____

❑ ____

B. **HOW TO HANDLE: Do not PUMP the shunt unless instructed by the neurosurgeon. Overpumping can drain the brain of fluid or cause other serious problems.**

____

____

____

____

____

____

____

____

____

____

____

____

____

____

____

____

____

8. ARNOLD CHIARI

❑ See additional sections with more information.

CONTACT 1. Primary caregiver ❑ See list ______________________________ Phone __________

2. Physician ❑ See list ____________________________________ Phone __________

➢ Notify the primary caregiver or the physician immediately if you notice an illness, condition, or an abnormality.

A. **SYMPTOMS. Your neurosurgeon will be able to give you more information for your individual condition.**

❑ ____

❑ ____

❑ ____

❑ ____

❑ ____

____

B. **HOW TO HANDLE. Seek medical attention immediately.**

____

____

____

____

____

____

____

____

____

____

____

____

____

9. ____

❑ <u>See additional sections with more information.</u>

<u>CONTACT</u> 1. Primary caregiver ❑ See list ______________________ Phone __________

2. Physician ❑ See list __________________________ Phone __________

➢ <u>Notify</u> the primary caregiver or the physician immediately if you notice an illness, condition, or an abnormality.

A. **SYMPTOMS**

❑ ____

❑ ____

❑ ____

❑ ____

❑ ____

B. **HOW TO HANDLE**

Medical Concerns Checklist Fill In

It will be important that all information is thoroughly documented and kept up to date. Separate fill-in section of this form is for you to customize to meet your needs.

MEDICAL CONCERNS CHECKLIST

Name____Date____________

CONTACT 1. Primary caregiver ❑ See list ___________________________ Phone __________

2. Physician ❑ See list _________________________________ Phone __________

➢ Notify the primary caregiver or the physician immediately if you notice an illness, condition, or an abnormality.

WHEN AN ILLNESS OR CONDITION OCCURS, HERE ARE AREAS TO CONSIDER.

There are separate sections regarding each area with more explicit information to assist you.

A. REMEMBER—if you need to go to the doctor or the emergency room, take the following:

a. *Personal Medical Journal* or *Medical History Summary*
b. Medical supply bag with the individual's specific incontinence and/or personal items, especially nonlatex items if there is a latex allergy.
c. *Personal Care Handbook* that includes specific personal information or the Medical Concerns Checklist.
d. Any X-rays to assist a medical professional that is located___________________________.

IMPORTANT: DO NOT LEAVE ANY X-RAYS OR REPORTS AT THE HOSPITAL OR AT PHYSICIAN'S OFFICE!

B. VOMITING. Always be alert for other symptoms that may be part of this situation.

a. ____
b. ____

C. BLOOD PRESSURE and HEART RATE

a. Normal is approximately 120/80. Individual's normal is__________________.
b. If elevated, check all areas in this Medical Concerns Checklist section for possible reasons for the elevation.

D. FEVER. Notify the primary caregiver and/or the physician immediately.

a. Individual's normal temperature is approximately_______________________.
b. Anything above normal warrants checking for a medical condition such as a urinary tract infection (UTI), decubitus, broken bones, infections, etc.

c. ____

E. CONCERN AREAS. The following areas have corresponding numbers to the pages that provides additional pertinent information:

1. ALLERGIES ❑ Medication ❑ Food ❑ ____________________ See Page______

2. DECUBITUS ____________________ See Page______

3. SEIZURES ____________________ See Page______

4. STROKE IDENTIFICATION ____________________ See Page______

5. URINARY TRACT INFECTION ____________________ See Page______

6. VOMITING ____________________ See Page______

7. SHUNTS ____________________ See Page______

8. ARNOLD CHIARI ____________________ See Page______

9. ____________________ See Page______

1. ALLERGIES

CONTACT 1. Primary caregiver ❑ See list ______________________________ Phone ___________

2. Physician ❑ See list ____________________________________ Phone ___________

➢ Notify the primary caregiver or the physician immediately if you notice an illness, condition, or an abnormality.

• **SEE MEDICATION AND FOOD ALLERGY LIST.** If additional information is needed, add another sheet.

i. **Medication** ❑ See additional list.

A. TYPE ____

1. Symptom ____
2. Remedy
   a. Medication ____
   b. How to assist ____
   c. ____

B. TYPE ____

1. Symptom ____
2. Remedy
   a. Medication ____
   b. How to assist ____
   c. ____

ii. **Foods** ❑ See additional list.

A. TYPE ____

1. Symptom ____
2. Remedy
   a. Medication ____
   b. How to assist ____
   c. ____

B. TYPE ____

1. Symptom ____
2. Remedy
   a. Medication ____
   b. How to assist ____
   c. ____

2. DECUBITUS, BEDSORES, BURNS

CONTACT 1. Primary caregiver ❑ See list ______________________________ Phone __________

2. Physician ❑ See list __________________________________ Phone __________

➢ Notify the primary caregiver or the physician immediately if you notice an illness, condition, or an abnormality.

• The physician will need to see the patient and may refer care to a wound care specialist.

A. Symptoms

a. ______________________________

b. ______________________________

c. ______________________________

d. ______________________________

B. Check body

a. ______________________________

b. ______________________________

c. ______________________________

d. ______________________________

e. ______________________________

f. ______________________________

g. ______________________________

h. ______________________________

C. Wounds

a. ______________________________

b. ______________________________

c. ______________________________

d. ______________________________

e. ______________________________

f. ______________________________

g. ______________________________

h. ______________________________

D. Cleaning of wound area

a. ______________________________

b. ______________________________

c. ______________________________

E. General information

a. ______________________________
b. ______________________________
c. ______________________________
d. ______________________________
e. ______________________________

F. Progression of wound healing generally observed. Check with the specialist for more information.

1. White layer
2. Pink layer
3. Bloody (good, means circulation is established)
4. Edges become smaller
5. Repeat of numbers 1–4 above until healed
6. Continually prompt and monitor to stay off the area.
7. Ask your physician if the following would be recommended:
   - Increased levels of zinc has been known to improve skin redevelopment. (Be sure to discuss with physician prior to increasing zinc so there is no conflict with treatment or medication. Zinc can be taken orally or used topically.)
   - Protein food or nutrients has been recognized as a good source for tissue redevelopment.

H. Travel. When going to the doctor or hospital, see Community Transportation, Section 6.

a. If you have latex allergies, take all nonlatex products in your medical travel bag with personal items, any applicable X-rays, and notebook or binder with caregiver notes, especially the Daily Vitals Record Keeping that includes the blood pressure and temperature.

I. Follow-up

a. ______________________________
____
b. ______________________________
____

J. Prevention techniques

a. Bedding: Monitor the bedding to ensure it is free of wrinkles and bulk, secured well, and the bottom area of the bedding is flat.
   - ______________________________
   - ______________________________

b. Cushions for wheelchairs and other seating devices.
    - Fitting is appropriate.
    - Placement is appropriate.

c. Cushion - Back
    - ______________________________
    - ______________________________

d. Cushion - Fabric
    - ______________________________
    - ______________________________

e. Cushion - Seating
    - ______________________________
    - ______________________________

f. Transfers: Watch how individual transfers in and out of chair.
    - ______________________________
    - ______________________________

3. SEIZURES

CONTACT 1. Primary caregiver ❑ See list ______________________________ Phone ___________

2. Physician ❑ See list ____________________________________ Phone ___________

➢ Notify the primary caregiver or the physician immediately if you notice an illness, condition, or an abnormality.

✶ **NOTE:** *Do not give* any Tylenol, aspirin, or ibuprofen-type medication. This can mask a symptom if there is a serious medical condition.

A. **Symptoms**

- ______________________________
- ______________________________
- ______________________________
- ______________________________

B. **Concerns**

- ______________________________
- ______________________________
- ______________________________

C. **Description of the seizures**

- ______________________________
- ______________________________
- ______________________________
- ______________________________
- ______________________________
- ______________________________

E. **During seizure concerns**

- ______________________________
- ______________________________
- ______________________________

D. **Follow-up**

- ______________________________
- ______________________________
- ______________________________
- ______________________________

E. Additional information

- ____________________
- ____________________
- ____________________

4. STROKE IDENTIFICATION

If he or she has trouble with ANY ONE of the following tasks, call emergency immediately and describe the symptoms to the dispatcher.

Sometimes symptoms of a stroke are difficult to identify. Unfortunately, the lack of awareness spells disaster. The stroke victim may suffer severe brain damage when people fail to recognize the symptoms of a stroke.

Now, doctors say YOU can recognize a stroke by asking three simple questions:

S - Ask the individual to SMILE.

T - Ask the person to TALK and SPEAK A SIMPLE SENTENCE (coherently) for example, "It is sunny out today" and person is unable to stay focused in the conversation.

R - Ask them to RAISE BOTH ARMS.

Another sign of a stroke: "Stick **O**ut Your Tongue"

- Ask the person to stick out his tongue.
- If the tongue is crooked or if it goes to one side or the other, that is also an indication of a stroke.

You may want to include additional information.

This is a situation that could have been prevented.

During a BBQ, a woman stumbled and took a little fall - she assured everyone that she was fine (they offered to call paramedics)...she said she had just tripped over a brick because of her new shoes.

They got her cleaned up and got her a new plate of food. While she appeared a bit shaken up, Jane went about enjoying herself the rest of the evening.

Jane's husband called later telling everyone that his wife had been taken to the hospital - (at 6:00 p.m. Jane passed away.) She had suffered a stroke at the BBQ.

Had they known how to identify the signs of a stroke, perhaps Jane would be with us today. Some don't die. They can end up in a helpless, hopeless condition instead.

A neurologist says that if he can get to a stroke victim within 3 hours he can totally hopefully reverse the effects of a stroke totally. He said the trick was getting a stroke recognized, diagnosed, and then getting the patient medically cared for within 3 hours, which can be the difficult part.

This information is to assist you and a collection from several sources.

5. URINARY TRACT INFECTION (UTI)

CONTACT 1. Primary caregiver ❑ See list ______________________________ Phone ___________

2. Physician ❑ See list ____________________________________ Phone ___________

➢ Notify the primary caregiver or the physician immediately if you notice an illness, condition, or an abnormality.

A. **SYMPTOMS**

a. ____

b. ____

c. ____

d. ____

e. ____

f. ____

g. ____

h. ____

B. **URINE ANALYSIS (UA)**

a. Doctor's office ____

b. Laboratory ____

c. How to obtain sample ____

- ____
- ____
- ____
- ____
- ____

C. **MAKE AN APPOINTMENT AS SOON AS POSSIBLE.**

a. Be sure to pack any incontinence products to include latex-free products if applicable.

- ____
- ____
- ____
- ____
- ____

D. **FOLLOW UP**. Find out if there is a bacterial infection and what treatment is recommended.

- ____
- ____
- ____
- ____

a. The doctor will give instructions as to what is needed, be sure to ask when the results will be available.

b. It will be important to follow up with a phone call or to check online for the results.

- Do not depend on a call back from the doctor's office.

c. If a prescription is necessary,

1. check against the allergy listing
2. give the doctor's office your pharmacy number or location
3. pick up the medication

d. When you pick up the medication, check to ensure it is what has been prescribed by the physician.

- ____
- ____
- ____
- ____

E. **RECHECK**. Be sure to ask the doctor if they need the following:

a. ____

1. Schedule follow-up appointment
2. Contact Outreach for transportation if applicable

F. **ADDITIONAL INFORMATION**

____

____

____

____

____

____

____

____

____

____

____

____

____

____

6. VOMITING

❑ This can be an indication of other concerns that need to be checked, such as the flu or another diagnosis.

CONTACT 1. Primary caregiver ❑ See list ______________________ Phone __________

2. Physician ❑ See list ______________________ Phone __________

➢ Notify the primary caregiver or the physician immediately if you notice an illness, condition, or an abnormality.

A. SYMPTOMS

a. Vomiting

1. Frequency ______________________

2. Color ❑ Food ❑ Blood ❑ Phlegm

3. ❑ Note ______________________

____

____

B. HOW TO HANDLE

❑ Call doctor ______________________

❑ Emergency Immediately ❑ Monitor ______________________

❑ Medication Type______________ Dosage__________ Frequency__________

❑ Other

____

____

____

____

____

____

____

____

____

____

____

____

____

7. SHUNTS

❑ See additional sections with more information.

CONTACT 1. Primary caregiver ❑ See list ______________________ Phone __________

2. Physician ❑ See list ____________________________ Phone __________

➤ Notify the primary caregiver or the physician immediately if you notice an illness, condition, or an abnormality.

A. **SYMPTOMS.** It will be best to list the symptoms you want to ensure that they are monitored by your physician.

❑ Headache ❑ Eye sensitivity to light ❑ Cognitive speech is unclear

❑ Red tracking on neck and chest areas ❑ Swelling around tubing area

❑ The ophthalmologist can check to see if there is pressure on the optic nerve.

❑ ____

❑ ____

❑ ____

❑ ____

B. **HOW TO HANDLE. Do not PUMP the shunt unless instructed by the neurosurgeon. Overpumping can drain the brain of fluid.**

____

____

____

____

____

____

____

____

____

____

____

____

____

____

8. ARNOLD CHIARI

❑ See additional sections with more information.

CONTACT 1. Primary caregiver ❑ See list ______________________________ Phone __________

2. Physician ❑ See list ____________________________________ Phone __________

➢ Notify the primary caregiver or the physician immediately if you notice an illness, condition, or an abnormality.

A. **SYMPTOMS. Your neurosurgeon will be able to give you more information for your individual condition.**

❑ ____

❑ ____

❑ ____

❑ ____

❑ ____

____

B. **HOW TO HANDLE. Seek medical attention immediately.**

____

____

____

____

____

____

____

____

____

____

____

____

____

____

For you to add additional medical concerns, make copies of this page for all areas.

9. ______________________________

❑ See additional sections with more information.

CONTACT 1. Primary caregiver ❑ See list ____________________ Phone __________

2. Physician ❑ See list ____________________ Phone __________

➢ Notify the primary caregiver or the physician immediately if you notice an illness, condition, or an abnormality.

A. **SYMPTOMS**

❑ ______________________________

❑ ______________________________

❑ ______________________________

❑ ______________________________

❑ ______________________________

B. **HOW TO HANDLE**

____

____

____

____

____

____

____

____

____

____

____

____

____

10
Medical Occurrence Log

- This form is used when a medical condition occurs to keep everyone abreast of a situation.
- To prevent future confusion, use one form per type of medical situation.
- This will maintain an independent frequency log of reoccurring events, such as urinary tract infections (UTIs), falls, seizures, etc.
- Take this with you to the doctor's office to show the frequency of a situation. This can assist your medical team to help find a diagnosis, the need for further testing, or medication to help prevent the occurrence of a specific problem.

Medical Occurrence Log

❑ ALLERGIES ❑ ________________ ❑ ________________
❑ OTHER ❑ ________________ ❑ ________________

- This can be used when there is a specific health occurrence and kept on a separate log form to assist a physician of the frequency.
- Always **document and alert** the primary caregiver or physician of a medical occurrence immediately.

DATE			
TIME			
TYPE (Allergy, seizure, etc.)			
EXPLAIN what occurred			
RX given			
REPORTED to			
REPORTED by			

11
Medication Daily Schedule and Chart

This is VERY IMPORTANT to keep up to date especially when medication needs to be distributed by the caregiver. It is recommended to have more than one pillbox for each time frame depending on the medication distribution. Having a medication pillbox will help in ensuring that the correct medication is taken and can prevent missing a medication, taking the wrong medication, or taking more than prescribed. It can be easy to forget you have taken a medication and then take another dosage.

You may want to keep the medication bottles in a separate container that holds all the medication along with the Medication Daily Schedule. This helps keep in them in a safe place, out of reach from visitors, and in some cases the person to whom they are prescribed as they may have a tendency to get into them; a person with cognitive issues or dementia can get confused and take their medication more than what is prescribed.

Keep a Medication Chart of all medication, over-the-counter, and herbal supplementals. It will be easier to stay aware of what and when medications have been taken, discontinued, or there was an allergy reaction.

Some pharmacies offer a 'Bubble Pak' type of system whereby they have all the medication separated by time. There could be an additional charge, but this is an alternative that you could ask your pharmacist.

As a caregiver of an individual requiring assistance, having a weekly medication tray is helpful to see if the medication has been taken and that the medication is set up correctly to avoid a mistake.

Be careful if you allow the individual who needs assistance to be in charge of the weekly medication pillbox. I recommend checking the pillbox to ensure that the medication is taken correctly. Also, if you have them fill the pillbox, watch and check that the medication is distributed correctly.

If a medication has been discontinued due to an allergic reaction, be sure to note it and add it to your "Allergy List." State what the reaction was and what medication or hospital emergency was needed to remedy the situation.

Medication Daily Schedule

Place the time and date in appropriate box.

Medication ______________________ Date started ______________________

Time

				Other

Discontinued Date__________ ❑ Monthly prescription refill Rx #______________

Reason: ❑ Completed ❑ Reaction: Be sure to add to Allergy Section - Medication.

Place the time and date in appropriate box.

Medication ______________________ Date started ______________________

Time

				Other

Discontinued Date__________ ❑ Monthly prescription refill Rx #______________

Reason: ❑ Completed ❑ Reaction: Be sure to add to Allergy Section - Medication.

Place the time and date in appropriate box.

Medication ______________________ Date started ______________________

Time

				Other

Discontinued Date__________ ❑ Monthly prescription refill Rx #______________

Reason: ❑ Completed ❑ Reaction: Be sure to add to Allergy Section - Medication.

Place the time and date in appropriate box.

Medication ______________________ Date started ______________________

Time

				Other

Discontinued Date__________ ❑ Monthly prescription refill Rx #______________

Reason: ❑ Completed ❑ Reaction: Be sure to add to Allergy Section - Medication.

Place the time and date in appropriate box.

Medication ______________________ Date started ______________________

Time

				Other

Discontinued Date__________ ❑ Monthly prescription refill Rx #______________

Reason: ❑ Completed ❑ Reaction: Be sure to add to Allergy Section - Medication.

Place the time and date in appropriate box.

Medication ______________________ Date started ______________________

Time

				Other

Discontinued Date__________ ❑ Monthly prescription refill Rx #______________

Reason: ❑ Completed ❑ Reaction: Be sure to add to Allergy Section - Medication.

Medication Chart

Keep a summary list of all medication even over-the-counter and herbal supplements, when discontinued, and specify if there was an allergy reaction.

Date	Medication	Purpose	Dosage & Frequency	Reaction	Stopped	Comments

12
Personal Bag Organization

This section helps to ensure that all personal bags for the individual who requires assistance has the information or items needed daily, in an emergency, or when traveling and to avoid an embarrassment because they didn't have the correct supplies when needed.

It will be important for the caregiver to check the bags periodically to ensure they have the appropriate items needed, such as a backpack with the daily personal supplies that may be needed if the individual must go to the bathroom or a doctor's appointment. If a person is incontinent, they may require items to ensure they maintain their dignity and avoid embarrassment of not being able to clean up when away from their home.

It may be helpful to have a second bag in the car when away all day as a backup. This helps ensure that if more supplies are used than usual, then there is always an emergency bag of supplies available.

Remember, for an individual who requires supplies, it is not easy to go to a store and purchase it, so having the items on hand makes it more comfortable and easier on everyone.

This section offers two (2) forms, one a sample explaining the form for quick reference for any items needed when leaving the home, and another for you to complete and customize to meet your needs.

Bag Organization

- Sample form for quick reference for any items needed when leaving the home.
- Separate fill-in section of this form for you to customize to meet your needs.

*SUPPLIES CAN VARY DEPENDING ON THE PERSONAL NEEDS.

I. MEDICATIONS

Pharmacy______________________________ **Phone**_______________

Location ____

❑ Pickup ❑ Delivery option available ❑ Bubble pack (check with pharmacist) ❑ _________

II. MEDICAL SUPPLIER. See supply list.

Name______________________________ **Phone**_______________

Delivery: ❑ Home delivery ❑ Pickup ❑ Auto ❑ Monthly ❑ Call frequency __________

❑ ____

III. BAG/CASE SUPPLIES

A. BACKPACK. This is to be attached to the back of the wheelchair or as a side bag for a walker, paying close attention to balance, ensuring that the weight of the bag does not cause instability.

1. Daily check and restock to ensure that it contains all necessary items.
2. All-day excursions may require more supplies. Some outings may require the following:
   a. Additional clothes in the event of an incontinence issue
   b. Personal supplies
   c. Additional cushion covers
   d. ____

B. HIP BAG/PURSE. Attached to wheelchair or walker.

1. This is the individual's responsibility; however, it may require the assistance of someone to ensure that they have what is needed.
2. For a female, it could be a purse; for a male, it could be a just a wallet in a small pack for additional items.
   a. Wallet with some type of identification and medical card.
   b. Other miscellaneous personal items.
   c. Cell phone, emergency phone numbers, etc.
   d. Extra medication needed while away from home; this may be also carried in the backpack.

C. HOSPITAL MEDICAL SUPPLY BAG/EMERGENCY BAG. Always take the Personal Medical Summary.

Located ______________________________

1. Used for any special medical supplies or personal items to ensure availability, keeping some of the hospital costs down.
    a. If a particular pair of briefs is used that helps reduce the incidence of a decubitus (the medical facility only has one type), the individual may want what fits properly and is comfortable.
    b. If there are allergies to certain materials such as latex, it is best to carry all latex-free items as not all hospitals or doctor offices have the same supplies.
    c. If there are ostomy supplies or catheters used, the size and product should be individualized. Taking your own supplies ensures you have what is needed at all times.
    d. Always bring your *Personal Medical Summary*, *Personal Medical Journal*, pertinent X-rays, and any medical, surgical, and/or laboratory reports to assist the medical team.

D. TRAVEL SUITCASE/BAG

Located ______________________________.

1. Always include current X-rays and *Personal Medical Summary* in case an emergency occurs.
2. Pack depending on the current medical needs and supplies.
3. Set out the clothes needed per day and include extra clothing and supplies should an incontinence event occur that will require additional changes.
4. Keep in mind whether or not you will need to do laundry while away; this will alter the number of items you are packing.

E. X-RAY CASE

Located ______________________________

1. Zipper art case holds X-rays nicely. You can purchase a case at the local art supply store.
2. **NEVER, NEVER, NEVER** allow the X-rays to stay at the hospital unless the physician has personal custody and they are being used for a procedure. This is personal history and critical for each physician to use in the different locations. They are critical to have when traveling in case of an emergency.
3. Take when you go to
    - ✓ emergency,
    - ✓ hospital,
    - ✓ procedure being considered, and
    - ✓ if needed for a doctor's appointment.

F. GROOMING/MAKEUP BAG

Located ____

1. Caregiver may handle or they may assist the individual.

Personal Bag Organization Fill In

- Sample form for quick reference for any items needed when leaving the home.
- Separate fill-in section of this form for you to customize to meet your needs.

*SUPPLIES CAN VARY DEPENDING ON THE PERSONAL NEEDS.

I. MEDICATIONS

Pharmacy____ **Phone**________________

Location____

❑ Pickup ❑ Delivery option available ❑ Bubble pack (check with pharmacist) ❑ __________

II. MEDICAL SUPPLIER. See supply list.

Name____ **Phone** ________________

Delivery: ❑ Home delivery ❑ Pickup ❑ Auto ❑ Monthly ❑ Call frequency ____________

❑ ____

III. BAG/CASE SUPPLIES

A. BACKPACK. Attached to back of wheelchair or a side bag for a walker, paying close attention to balance and ensuring the weight of the bag does not cause instability.

1. ____
2. ____
3. ____
4. ____

B. HIP BAG/PURSE. Attached to wheelchair or walker.

This is the individual's responsibility; however, it may require the assistance of someone to ensure that they have what is needed.

1. ____
2. ____
3. ____
4. ____

C. HOSPITAL MEDICAL SUPPLY BAG/EMERGENCY BAG. Always take your *Personal Medical Summary.*

Located ____

Used for any special medical supplies or personal items to ensure availability, keeping some of the hospital costs down.

1. ____

2. ______________________________
3. ______________________________
4. ______________________________

D. TRAVEL SUITCASE/BAG

Located ______________________________

1. ______________________________
2. ______________________________
3. ______________________________
4. ______________________________
5. ______________________________
6. ______________________________

E. X-RAY CASE

Located ______________________________

1. Black zipper art case holds X-rays nicely. You can purchase a case at the local art supply store.
2. **NEVER, NEVER, NEVER** allow the X-rays to stay at the hospital unless the physician has personal custody and they are being used for a procedure. This is personal history and critical for each physician to use in the different locations. They are critical to have when traveling in case of an emergency.
3. ______________________________
4. ______________________________
5. ______________________________
6. ______________________________

F. GROOMING/MAKEUP BAG

Located ______________________________

1. ______________________________
2. ______________________________
3. ______________________________
4. ______________________________
5. ______________________________
6. ______________________________

13
Personal Medical Summary

Using this form provides a medical history summary that should be shown to your physician at each visit and especially the emergency team so they can be sure of the medical history you have. The physicians today must move quickly between each patient so that by providing your medical summary, it can assist them; even if all the information is in the computer, this helps simplify and provide a quick resource of invaluable information that you can refer to and remind them if need be.

Physicians even in medical facilities that have everything computerized find this form extremely helpful and utilize it; it shows you care about your health, and they appreciate it.

When traveling, this offers you the information in the event you need to seek medical assistance.

It is important to summarize your past and current health information.

- If you are unable to recall the exact date, use the approximate year.
- Surgeries and procedures—if you do not remember the exact name, give a brief explanation.
- Complete as much history as you can remember, and feel free to include all pertinent information that will be helpful during an emergency or medical treatment.
- Be sure to update as needed at least every six (6) months to ensure that the information is correct. Sometimes a medication is changed, and this way, you will have the current information.
- If you have an emergency and unable to speak for yourself, this will help the person assisting you to ensure that the medical team has your up-to-date information.
- Make copies of your summary and keep a current master for your files. Take a picture of it and send it to your cell phone for a copy, and keep a copy as well in your book bag.

Personal Medical Summary

Keep this summary updated and present it to your medical/dental professional at all visits.

<table>
<tr><td colspan="4">Name (Last, First, M.I.)</td><td>☐ M ☐ F</td><td colspan="3">DOB</td></tr>
<tr><td>Marital status</td><td colspan="7">E-mail address</td></tr>
<tr><td colspan="3">Address</td><td colspan="3">City</td><td>ST</td><td>Zip</td></tr>
<tr><td>Phone</td><td colspan="3">Fax</td><td colspan="2">Mobile</td><td colspan="2">Work</td></tr>
<tr><td>SS no. Xxx-xx-</td><td>Blood Type</td><td>Religion</td><td colspan="5">Mother's maiden name</td></tr>
<tr><td colspan="2">Nearest relative</td><td>Phone</td><td colspan="5">Relationship</td></tr>
</table>

Medications Currently Taking

☐ See attached sheet for more information.

	Date	Drug	Dosage	Amount	Frequency	Purpose
1.						
2.						
3.						
4.						
5.						
6.						
7.						
8.						
9.						
10.						

Instructions

PURPOSE: To assist your medical/dental provider with your current up-to-date information for their files and to ensure that their information is current.

The Personal Medical Summary is to complement your Personal Medical Journal. Use as a condensed summary of your personal medical history. Take your Personal Medical Journal with you to the appointment and update the summary as needed.

Suggestions:

1. Before filling out forms, make extra copies to ensure availability of more forms to update as needed.
2. Be sure to take your Personal Medical Summary with you to all appointments that may need your medical history, including schools.
3. Take a copy with you when traveling to ensure you have the information you may need at your fingertips in the event you become ill or have an emergency.

Although the author has made every effort to ensure the accuracy and completeness of information contained in this form, she assumes no responsibility for errors, inaccuracies, omissions, or any inconsistency herein.

For more information or to order replacement forms, contact **Life Cycles Publishing Inc.** at PO Box 41122, San Jose, CA 95160, www.lcpbooks.com or info@lcpbooks.com

Name ______________________________

Allergies <u>Medications</u>

☐ See attached sheet for more information.

	Date	**Medication**	**Reaction**	**Counterapplication** (What did you take or do to relieve the allergy?)
1.				
2.				
3.				
4.				
5.				
6.				
7.				
8.				
9.				
10.				

➢ **<u>Note</u>:** Generic Rx products ☐ Yes ☐ No

Allergies <u>Foods</u>

	Date	**Food**	**Reaction**	**Counterapplication** (What did you take or do to relieve the allergy?)
1.				
2.				
3.				
4.				
5.				
6.				
7.				
8.				
9.				
10.				

Name ______________________________

Medical Conditions Diagnosis

☐ See attached sheet for more information.

	Date	Diagnosis	Problem	Comment
1.				
2.				
3.				
4.				
5.				
6.				
7.				
8.				
9.				
10.				

Alerts or Medical Illnesses

Health notation: Something you and/or your doctor/therapist are watching or monitoring.

☐ See attached sheet for more information.

	Date	Physician	Description	Concerns/Comment
1.				
2.				
3.				
4.				
5.				
6.				
7.				
8.				
9.				
10.				

Name ______________________________

Surgeries/Hospitalizations

☐ See attached sheet for more information.

	Date	Hospital, City, State	Procedure	Comment
1.				
2.				
3.				
4.				
5.				
6.				
7.				
8.				
9.				
10.				

Tests, X-Rays, Procedures

☐ See attached sheet for more information.

	Date	Hospital, City, State	Procedure	X-ray	Purpose	Results
1.						
2.						
3.						
4.						
5.						
6.						
7.						
8.						
9.						
10.						

Name ______________________________

Family History

	Date	Diagnosis	Relative	Comment
1.				
2.				
3.				
4.				
5.				

➢ PLEASE NOTE IMPORTANT INFORMATION THAT HAS NOT BEEN STATED.

____

____

____

____

____

____

____

____

____

Immunizations

Date	Physician	Immunization	Next Due	Purpose	Reactions
		Tetanus			
		Influenza			
		Pneumonia			
		MMR *Measles, Mumps, Rubella*			

Name ______________________________

Physicians, Dentist, Service Providers

	Date	Name	Address, City, State, Zip	Phone	Specialty

Insurance Information

Medical Provider/s ____________________ ____________________ ____________________

Medical No. ______________________ Other Hospital No. ____________ ____________

Medicare No. __________________ Medi-Cal/State Provider No.______________________

Other ____

Subscriber ________________________________ Subscriber No.______________________

Effective ____

Member Services Phone No. (____)______________ (____)______________ (____)______________

Deductible $ _______ Co Pay $ ________ Office Visit $ ________ Hospital $ _________

Emergency $ _________ Out of Service/Plan Area $ _________ Other $ ____________________

Medication: Generic $ ________________ Non-Generic $ _______________

Name ______________________________

Primary Physician ______________________________
Plan Code ______________________________
Employer ______________________________
Address ______________________________
Phone (____) ______________________________

Dentist______________________________
Carrier ______________________________
Plan Code ________ Check with the doctor office or plan administrator regarding the fee schedule.

Other Coverage______________________________
Carrier ______________________________
Plan Code _________Check with the doctor office or plan administrator regarding the fee schedule.

NOTES ☐ See attached sheet.

____
____
____
____
____
____
____
____
____
____
____
____
____
____
____
____

➢ Add a separate page for any notes you feel are important regarding your health that you want to ensure your medical/dental team are informed.

14
Endorsement and Other Publications Available

ENDORSEMENT

Ms. Lopez would appreciate your endorsement. Please complete the attached endorsement sheet and return as stated on the form.

OTHER PUBLICATIONS AVAILABLE

A list of other publications is listed. Return the completed form for more information or additional copies.

Ms. Lopez is always available as a speaker at your organization or a meeting. Call to schedule a time to hear her and the wonderful wealth of information that she offers.

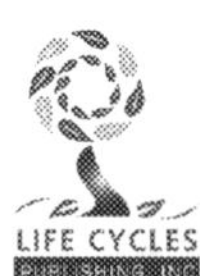

LIFE CYCLES PUBLISHING, INC.

P.O. Box 41122, San Jose, CA 95160 –www.lcpbooks.com

RE: ENDORSEMENT

As you are a valued individual, I would appreciate if you would consider providing me with your endorsement regarding the importance of maintaining your personal medical history to eliminate medical errors.

❑ All ❑ Personal Medical Journal ❑ My Personal Medical Journal ❑ Personal Medical Pocket Journal

❑ Personal Care Handbook ❑ Personal Caregiver Handbook

Please keep your comment brief, preferably to 1–3 lines.

____

____

____

How would you want your name to appear?

Name ________________________________

Title ________________________________

Business ________________________________

Other ________________________________

I give permission to use the above statement in the following:

- ❑ All Literature, to include
  - ❑ books, either on the front or back cover and not limited within the text content
- ❑ Web site, Internet
- ❑ Social media ❑ All ❑ Except ________________________
- ❑ Newspapers, magazines, periodicals
- ❑ I would like to be kept informed when my name will be applied to anything.
- ❑ I want to limit this endorsement to the following: ____________________

  ____

  ____

Signed______________________________Date____________

Phone__________________________E-mail________________

Please either	Mail this to	Life Cycles Publishing P.O. Box 41122 San Jose, CA 95160	E-mail:	Info@lcpbooks.com

Should you have any questions, please do not hesitate to contact me.

In appreciation,

Gloria Lopez, CEO/Author

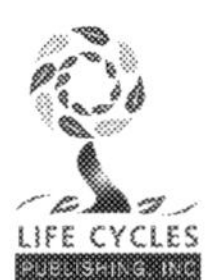

LIFE CYCLES PUBLISHING, INC

P.O. Box 41122, San Jose, CA 95160 –www.lcpbooks.com

Books available from Life Cycles Publishing Inc. and Author Gloria Lopez for purchase

The following items are available for purchase individually and in bulk.

Consider giving this as a gift that will further aid your clients. Call us to find out more regarding customizing the cover to include your business name.

They can provide you or your clients the opportunity to maintain personal medical history, eliminating memorization and medical errors through documentation. It also provides the tools needed when working with various professionals.

❒ Personal Medical Journal Spiral-bound 254-page self-help journal

Maintains an individual's personal medical history from pregnancy and throughout their lifetime.

❒ My Personal Medical Journal ❒ Hard cover ❒ Soft cover 230-page self-help journal

Maintains an individual's personal medical history throughout their lifetime.

❒ Personal Medical Pocket Journal 3.5″ × 7″ self-help journal 32 pages

A condensed pocket summary of an individual's health history.
Easy to carry in a purse or pocket.

❒ Personal Care Handbook

Provides an individual with a chronic medical condition requiring the assistance of a caregiver to explain in detail their medical needs, explaining the disability, medical concerns, all medical supplies needed, and how to hire a caregiver.

❒ Personal Caregiver Handbook

Used daily by a caregiver with instructions and a variety of daily charting forms depending on the individual needs to assist in monitoring their health. The charts can be a helpful tool to take to the doctor's appointment.

❒ Food Allergy Card

Used to present to waitresses and/or chefs to notify them of food allergies the person may have toward specific foods and spices.

- ✓ Eliminate potential cross contamination, allowing the restaurant to prepare the food safely.
- ✓ Cards will be customized to include your company logo.

❒ I am interested in more information and the possibility of purchasing. Please check the above books of interest.

Name ______________________________ Title______________

Company ____

Phone ____________________ E-mail____________________

Printed in the United States
By Bookmasters